CHALLENGING THE ANXIOUS BRAIN

A PRACTICAL GUIDE FOR ANXIOUS PEOPLE.
INCLUDES AN ACTIONABLE 7-DAY PLAN TO MANAGE
ANXIOUS PEAKS.

TORI WARNER

CONTENTS

INTRODUCTION

My first experience with anxiety was when I was twenty-five years old. I was living in London after a year spent traveling the world and I had landed a great new job in sales. I had moved into a beautiful new flat with my boyfriend and I was ready to do fully-fledged adulting. Life should have been good. It should have been a hedonistic time of socializing with friends and enjoying the regular paycheck that I had missed for so long. But, that wasn't to be my reality. I wasn't sure what triggered that first panic attack, but after much searching and trying to figure it out, I now know it was driven by my anxious brain.

In retrospect, I can see the main problem was transitioning, overnight, from living out of a backpack, spending my days sitting on a beach, to a daily tube commute, rent to pay and a job with high sales targets. The shock of going from one world to another resulted in a spectacular panic attack!

I was walking home from work one evening when I suddenly felt my chest tighten, my heart beating so hard I thought it would be visible from the outside. My vision blurred and sounds became deafeningly loud. All I could focus on was getting back to the flat so I could call an ambulance to save me from the *heart attack* I was obviously having. Even in that moment, I knew rationally that at twenty-five it couldn't possibly be the case that I was having a heart attack but the physical symptoms were so intense, I really did feel like I was dying. Right then and there. My boyfriend called an ambulance and the paramedics, who were wonderful, tried their best to reassure me I was not about to die and what I was feeling was a *panic attack*. Their advice? Breathe and relax. Oh, how simple they made it sound... And there started my beautiful relationship with anxiety.

I am now forty-five, and I've not had a panic attack for over fifteen years. I've worked hard to understand the anatomy and chemical reliance of the brain, and I've explored how holistic approaches such as meditation, counseling and reiki can soothe the anxious brain. I want to pass on what I've learned so that it can help you too.

Although I'm not a doctor or a neuroscientist, I do have first-hand knowledge of what it's like to live with an anxious brain – and how to move through periods of anxiety. In some instances, I've even found ways to be grateful for the anxiety.

Bear with me, you might have achieved the same by the end of this book.

For me, anxiety was debilitating and sometimes paralyzing. While anxiety is a frightening experience, I want you to know that it is fixable and not something you have to endure. With understanding, practical advice and commitment to change, you can combat those debilitating feelings and live with personal compassion, anxiety-free.

You may feel you have tried *everything* to overcome your anxiety and nothing works! I really hope you read this book with an open mind and a willingness to change. Practice the methods without judgment. Read the explanations with curiosity. Look at yourself in a different light and say 'this will get better.' To live without anxiety, you need to approach your mental health with welcoming, compassion, and understanding.

To start, let's try to answer, 'what the heck is anxiety anyway?'

WHAT THE HECK IS ANXIETY ANYWAY?

In this chapter, we will explore:

- What anxiety is
- Types of anxiety disorders
- Potential causes of anxiety
- The importance of triggers
- Nature VS Nurture
- Trauma and grief anxiety

During those first anxious periods in my life, I remember feeling terrified. Not just of the panic attacks and the other debilitating symptoms, but also the feeling I was 'going crazy'.

My feelings were so intense, I had a really hard time rationalizing what was happening, and therefore the only conclusion I could come to was that I was going insane. I would sit for hours contemplating every intrusive thought, every muscle twitch, every jitter of my hands, and how they must mean I was losing my mind. This was utterly terrifying and gave even more power and energy to my anxiety.

After my first child was born, my anxiety found a whole new sphere to work its magic in. Not only was I anxious for myself, but I was now also anxious about her and my ability to look after her! I'd had no idea of the crushing responsibility I would feel by actually becoming a Mom. I was anxious that my anxiety would stop me from loving her, and looking after her 'properly'. In addition to these worries, having a newborn has a huge impact on our sleeping patterns, so I was torn between desperately wanting to sleep and being too afraid to sleep in case she needed me. My anxiety robbed me of those precious first weeks with my new baby girl. But I also learned a lot during that period. I learned self-compassion, patience, and most helpfully, what was happening biologically in my body.

Understanding what was happening biologically and neurochemically gave me confidence in my ability to control my thoughts, feelings, and, ultimately, my anxiety.

[1]**WHAT IS ANXIETY?**

[2]Have you ever crossed the road, and some driver almost runs you over because they didn't see the red light? Or perhaps you have sat watching television, and out of nowhere, you hear a loud bang coming from outside your window? In both

examples, your heart races, you start to sweat, you begin to shake, you may even feel nauseous, and your thoughts are going a mile a minute. This all happens within a matter of seconds until you realize the danger is over, then you quickly return to normal.... Or you don't. This feeling is anxiety. Every person on this planet experiences some level of anxiety. It's what keeps us alive and motivates us to stay away from danger. However, for some of us, these feelings of worry and fear become too extreme and prolonged. They overload our systems and sometimes pop up out of nowhere without any obvious cause. This is when anxiety is no longer a straightforward safety mechanism and is often referred to as Anxiety Disorder.

TYPES OF ANXIETY DISORDERS

There are many types of anxiety disorders. Although I am not a physician or medical practitioner myself, I know that if you have felt what I have for more than six weeks, you should definitely see a doctor to get a clinical diagnosis. However, you may already know you have an anxiety disorder, and that is why you are here. Anxiety comes in various forms and is not the same for everyone, but these are some of the more common types of anxiety:

- Generalized Anxiety Disorder (GAD)
- Panic disorder
- Phobias

○ Agoraphobia
○ Claustrophobia (Afraid of small spaces)
○ Arachnophobia (Afraid of spiders)
○ Acrophobia (Afraid of heights)

- Social Anxiety Disorder (Social Phobia)
- Obsessive-Compulsive Disorder (OCD)
- Post-Traumatic Stress Disorder (PTSD)
- Medication-induced Anxiety (Irrational fear of drugs)

POTENTIAL CAUSES OF ANXIETY

[3]Factors such as stress, personal relationships, health issues, financial concerns and lack of sleep can all contribute to increased anxiety. Years of medical and academic research have shown that no one knows the ultimate cause of anxiety disorders, and there is very rarely just one cause. However, we do know anxiety levels can be influenced by the way we live our lives and by our behaviors. We may sometimes avoid a situation because previously it has caused an anxious response, which then makes us believe, 'If I avoid that situation, my panic won't happen again'. This way of thinking is a completely understandable coping mechanism, but it can make anxiety worse and encourage patterns of anxious thought.

UNDERSTANDING THE IMPORTANCE OF TRIGGERS

[4]Often, we look to identify what triggers our anxiety and start to search for solutions to avoid them. It is important to have the right knowledge at the start of our journey for solutions, and the first step is to take an in-depth look at our triggers.

At the beginning of this chapter, I shared a story of my personal experience fighting postnatal anxiety. How it filled me with distressing thoughts and made me question my ability to really be a mother. I was filled with questions like, would I be too anxious to take care of her? What if she needed me in the night, but I couldn't help her because I was asleep? This led me to solve these 'problems' by staying awake – always! During the night when I was awake and flooded with anxiety, my mind would race with other potential threats to my daughter and how I could avoid them. It was crushing and utterly exhausting.

Although I got through this period, it stole the precious time I had of just *being* with my baby girl. Can you see how questioning and obsessing can create even more anxiety? My primary motivation was not just for myself but for my daughter, so it was especially important for me to find answers.

Part of understanding triggers is finding the inspiration for where to start healing. Identifying and understanding triggers is just one part of the puzzle.

There are also biological factors and our learned behavior

that adds to our anxious mind. Are we born anxious? Or is it something we learn? In essence, is it nature vs. nurture?

NATURE VS NURTURE

Have you asked yourself – as I have – 'is anxiety genetic?' 'Was I born this way?'

[5]Anxiety disorder can sometimes have a genetic component, but it is not an automatic outcome of having an anxious parent. Equally, growing up in a highly-stressful environment doesn't necessarily render you anxious.

Biological

[6]There are biological reasons why some people are more susceptible to anxiety. This does not mean that you are born with anxiety or that anxiety is a core element of who you are, and neither does it mean that it's something you have to just learn to live with. It merely means some people are more sensitive to an anxious response than others. Once we learn to recognize the physical sensations of anxiety, we can train ourselves to respond differently.

Biologically, one theory for the cause of anxiety is a hormone or chemical imbalance. For example, someone may have too much cortisol (the stress hormone) in their body. Or, have too little serotonin, the hormone responsible for our feelings of contentment. Always speak to a doctor about these concerns and never self-diagnose.

Learned behavior

It can be controversial to say anxiety is learned, but I think this can be quite reassuring. After all, anything that is learned can be changed. Neuroscientists talk of neural plasticity, which is how the brain grows and changes to create new pathways of thinking. Basically, it is possible to interrupt the brain's default way of thinking and change it for the better – or not.

For example, if we feel anxious in a grocery store, we devise an escape plan for if we start to feel panicky. We make a mental note of where the exits are, and while shopping, we reroute the escape. But then something unexpected happens, such as running into a talkative friend. Our body reacts out of fear that we can't escape and runs at an increased speed of thought trying to find other options of escape. Now, eventually, everything works out, and we leave the store. But if this continues to happen every time we go to the store, the brain says, 'oh, this is inevitable. Every time I go out, this happens, so I might as well stay home, so it doesn't happen again'. This is how we learn an anxiety behavior pattern.

My father suffered from anxiety and depression throughout my childhood. This was never talked about in the home, and it wasn't something I was aware of until my late teens, but looking back, I can see how the anxious brain of my twenties made me behave in very similar ways to him. I became obsessed with routine and completely intolerant of noise, exactly like he was. I had learned his 'coping mechanisms' for anxiety and was using them because they were all I had to work with! Who knows how different things would have been for both of us had anxiety been talked about and understood in the 1980s as it is now.

So, while many factors cause anxiety, it often creates a [7]vicious cycle in our minds. First, we get anxiety symptoms; next, we find an unhealthy way to escape the feelings and resolve the symptoms, then we gain relief and make a mental note of how to avoid it happening again. This all contributes to learning long-term negative behavior patterns. But it doesn't have to be this way. Once we identify our anxieties, even if we don't wholly understand them or our triggers, we can work on learning how to break our negative patterns.

TRAUMA AND GRIEF AS A CAUSE OF ANXIETY

[8]Post-Traumatic Stress Disorder is when an individual experiences anxiety because a traumatic memory has surfaced due to a current life event. For example, we may experience panic when we hear yelling, slamming doors, or loud noises. Or, we may experience anxiety when we witness someone else going through a similar experience we have had. Perhaps you are watching a movie, and you watch something that triggers a traumatic memory, and now you're experiencing some form of panic and anxiety. This is trauma-induced anxiety. However, just because we become anxious when our trauma has been triggered, it does not necessarily mean we now have PTSD. Post-Traumatic Stress Disorder evolves when the trauma in our lives starts to take over. Meaning it starts to control how

we live our daily lives. Some symptoms that accompany PTSD are:

- Daily flashbacks
- Distressing bodily sensations when reminded of the trauma
- Reliving trauma (envisioning it, which causes anxiety-like symptoms)
- Obsessive thoughts about the past
- Recurring nightmares based on the trauma

Trauma usually comes from something that has happened in your past, but some people have difficulty identifying where the trauma begins and where it ends. Because of this, you may not always know where the trauma is coming from.

GRIEF

Grief is incredibly painful and is a personal journey that is different for everyone and unfortunately something we all experience in our lives. However, usually, the journey of grief does get easier over time and we begin to feel hope and joy again as time passes. Grief happens in stages and anxiety is one stage that is normal in the grieving process. But when we find ourselves continuing to be in this anxious state over a long period of time, the anxiety is acting as a habit that is unavoidable.

An anxiety disorder that stems from grief is sustained and

unmoving. When we experience grief, we may become afraid of our emotions following a mournful event such as a loved one passing away or going through a divorce or break-up. For example, your child goes off to college, you may have an empty feeling and go into mourning. This phase in life is normal, and leading up to the event, we may feel some symptoms of anxiety such as, nervousness, nausea, dissociation, and an uncomfortable feeling of change. However, the feeling should pass within a short matter of time once you become used to your child being away, once you realize that they aren't really gone. On the other hand, if these anxious feelings continue, and we stay stuck in the grieving process of the life event, we may start to experience feelings of anxiety surrounding our emotions – especially if we cannot control your feelings anymore.

[9]For many, grief happens in stages which is normal, however, anxiety in grief can last for much too long, resulting in avoidance behavior or withdrawal from ourselves and others. This is anxiety in grief. You cannot take pleasure from anything and your mood refuses to lift regardless, possibly turning into depression. Anxiety is then triggered by the relentless feeling of hopelessness for the future. Again it is incredibly important to seek help for grief, whether that be taking therapy or medicinal help.

When exploring the reasons for our anxiety we inevitably ask; Why do *I* have anxiety? Did I cause it? Why am I so weak? If you take nothing else away from this book, know this, you are not to 'blame' for your anxiety and you are absolutely not weak!

CHAPTER SUMMARY

In this chapter, we looked at the different types of anxiety disorders, why they become a disorder, and the importance of finding our triggers. Now we have a deeper understanding of what anxiety is, we can start resolving it healthily.

Remember:

- Anxiety is not something you have to grit your teeth and live through.
- The anxious mind can be changed to react in more appropriate ways to serve our lives better.
- Anxiety is not 'your fault'!

2

BASIC (AND I MEAN BASIC) BRAIN BIOLOGY

In this chapter, we will look to understand:

- The parts of the brain and nervous system that effect anxiety.
- What happens in the brain during an anxiety attack
- How we can calm the anxious brain
- Actions to take to strengthen our resilience to anxiety

The physical symptoms of an anxious brain can be, at best frustrating, and at worst debilitating. It is hard to remember when we are feeling anxious that the symptoms will pass and are only temporary. It is that feeling of relentlessness that I

personally found so difficult. I desperately wanted to understand 'when it would end'.

The anxious brain and the physical symptoms we feel are
created by a mixture of anatomy, hormones, and brain
messengers (neurotransmitters). For me, it helped to understand the biology of what was happening inside me and why I
was feeling so bombarded by my mind and body. I needed to
take away the mystery of my anxiety and understand, in a very
basic way, what was going on biologically.

Once I understood the biology and why my body was
reacting the way it was, I felt much more empowered to take
back control. It helped me become less frustrated by my feelings and emotions and more rational in responding to them. I
found compassion for myself in knowing my brain and body
were trying to help me survive and not trying to sabotage my
life. Understanding what each physical symptom was and why
it occurred meant I could respond objectively rather than
panicking to make it 'go away!' It meant I could counteract
the unpleasant physical symptoms or accept them and wait for
them to pass independently. I decided to go with the flow
rather than fight it.

I used to have incredible nausea when I was anxious. It
would seemingly come from nowhere, and I really felt like I
was going to vomit. I never did, by the way. However, in
response to nausea, I wouldn't eat for fear of making it worse
or actually making myself vomit. As a result, my body would
respond by thinking, 'aha, there must be something wrong

because now we have no food and therefore no energy source,' so the anxiety symptoms would increase.

I learned that by eating something, nausea would slowly go away, and the anxiety would reduce. I don't mean I would eat a whole meal in one sitting, but I would eat small amounts and often, every two hours or so. Foods that I found helped were:

- a slice of toast and half a chopped apple
- plain biscuit with a slice of cheese
- toasted English muffin with peanut butter or jam
- a slice of chicken and some grapes

At this point, I feel it is important to reiterate, I am not a doctor or neuroscientist, and so this chapter is my layman's interpretation of the workings of the anxious brain. I genuinely believe it is crucial to understand how and why the anxious brain behaves, in order to change the patterns and reactions we have that are harming us.

Remember, the brain's primary purpose is to keep us alive! It just wants to process incoming data and make predictions of how to respond to ensure our survival. It has no moral obligation to make us happy or sad.

THE BRAIN

Firstly, let's look at 2 parts of the brain that are critical to our anxious responses:

· · ·

1 The Amygdala

[1]The amygdala is a small area near the base of the brain. There are actually two amygdalae, one on each side. They are pretty small – about the size of walnuts – but incredibly important in processing our emotions.

The amygdala is where our emotions are given meaning, associations, and remembered for the future. It is particularly vital in processing strong emotions such as fear and pleasure. I find it useful to think of the amygdala as our brains' 'first responder'. It is incredibly reactive and is continuously scanning the world to identify threats. The amygdala evolved to improve our chances of survival by initiating the infamous fight-or-flight response.

What Happens in The Brain During An Anxiety Attack

Once the amygdala identifies a potential threat, it sends messages to the body to prepare to run away or stand and fight the danger. Either response requires your body to be flooded with hormones to get you into a heightened state and focus entirely on the impending threat. The amygdala can make this happen almost instantaneously, before the rest of your brain has time to process the situation.

Sounds like a good, stable system, right? The problem is that the world has evolved at a lightning pace compared to our biological evolution and so what the amygdala senses is not always reliable. It is totally appropriate to be anxious (terrified) about a lion stalking you, and you definitely want your amygdala to hit the 'let's get out of here now' button. However, the amygdala doesn't know how to respond differently when you become agitated about a notification pinging to tell you there is a meeting you are late for. Remember, your brain is only interested in your survival, so it is not going to take any chances. It would rather over-prepare than die!

2 PREFRONTAL CORTEX (PFC)

Our prefrontal cortex (PFC) is the most evolved part of our brains and is responsible for rational thinking, decision-making, and planning. However, because the amygdala is our first responder and literally eavesdrops on all of our senses, it is ready to jump into action before our PFC has time to process any danger. The amygdala is super fast and will hit the fight-or-flight button before your PFC has a chance to catch up. This is useful if a lion is stalking you. You don't need your thinking brain to process the danger and decide what to do. You need to get the heck out of there!

However, an overzealous amygdala initiates a life-or-death response to even non-threatening situations. Your PFC thinking brain doesn't stand a chance of stepping in, assessing the situation, and responding in a moderated way.

Actions to Take: [2]**How to Calm The amygdala and Help The PFC Take The Lead**

Stop! Count

First things first, stop and evaluate your situation. When your mind (amygdala) tells you to run, look out, and hide, it's sending you physical symptoms so that you can act immediately. If you pay attention to your surroundings, rather than what your physical symptoms are doing, you're choosing to think with your rational mind (Prefrontal-Cortex). So, stop and count to ten slowly to let your PFC engage. We will be looking at these strategies in more detail in chapter six.

Meditate or Breathe

When your mind is running at a thousand miles a minute, it is hard to focus. After you have stopped and counted to ten, take a seat and breathe. You can try a quick exercise called Boxed Breathing.

- Breathe in for 4 seconds
- Hold for 4 seconds
- Breathe out for 4 seconds
- And repeat.

Once these breathing steps have taken place, your symptoms should start to slow down because you are consciously telling your amygdala there is no threat here. You may become dizzy, so don't force your breath, and after a few rounds of *box breathing,* do start to breathe normally. Or try *diaphragmatic breathing:*

- Put one hand on your chest and one hand on your stomach.
- When you breathe in, your belly should be pushing your hand up while your chest hand remains still.
- Once this becomes a pattern, focus deeply on your breath. Push your thoughts aside (for now) and focus on your breath:

  - Where is your breath coming from? Nose, stomach, lungs?
  - What does it feel like? Cold, warm, body temperature?
  - Notice your breath and visualize its color. Is it red for angry, blue for calm, or green for neutral?

This is a form of meditation, a great strategy for beating anxiety that we will talk more about in chapter six. Once we are relaxed and our bodily sensations have slowed, we can work on figuring out what caused the anxious response in the first place.

Challenge Your Thoughts

After the anxiety has passed, ask yourself; what were you feeling at that exact moment? What is your emotional mind telling you as opposed to your rational mind?

Try asking yourself:

What triggered my senses?

- Why is my skin tingly?
- Why is my heart racing?
- I heard a sound I'm unsure of
- I've entered an unfamiliar place

What is my amygdala telling me?

- Skin sensations = There must be something wrong
- Racing heartbeat = It's time to be scared. Let's run. Get out of here
- Unfamiliar noise = Don't investigate, hold your breath, and hide
- My surroundings don't make sense = RUN! You are in danger

How realistic is my amygdala being? Listen to your prefrontal cortex.

- Bodily sensations = PFC says 'I'm cold' vs. Amygdala: 'New symptom, something is up'

- Racing heart = PFC says 'A normal response to my situation' vs. Amygdala: 'Run'
- Unfamiliar noise = PFC says 'It was a ball dropping/ the house settling/ the sink dripping/ etc' vs. Amygdala: 'Hide'
- Unfamiliar surroundings = PFC says 'New experiences lead to greater comfort zones. Let's just chill.' vs. Amygdala: 'I need to get out of here. Nothing makes sense. DANGER'

Can you see the difference? By paying attention to what your emotional mind (Amygdala) is telling you and listening to your rational mind (Prefrontal Cortex), you are attaching positive memories to your anxiety triggers and sensations. If you continue to do this every time you have anxiety or have been triggered, it will become second-nature down the road when your amygdala wants to tell you there is danger, but there is none. Essentially, you are rewiring and retraining your amygdala to re-evaluate what's dangerous and what isn't. That way, when you really are in danger, your amygdala will be able to do its job more efficiently, thus getting you out of a challenging situation when you need it.

THE VAGUS NERVE

Controlling the inner nervous system, the vagus nerve is the longest cranial nerve, connecting the brain, major organs and colon. It is also often referred to as the 'chillout nerve', able to decrease alertness, blood pressure, and heart rate. It can promote calmness and relaxation throughout the body.

When our fight-or-flight response kicks in and floods us with stress hormones, the vagus nerve releases helpful chemicals like acetylcholine and oxytocin, which, among other things, calm us down. This is called the [3]*vagal tone*. If it is too low, our ability to regulate and handle stress becomes compromised because the vagal tone is responsible for emotional response.

Multiple studies have shown that by increasing and strengthening the vagal tone, we will be more likely to recover more quickly after stress, injury, or illness.

Actions to Take to Calm The Vagus Nerve

[4]How to activate and strengthen the Vagus Nerve

- **Cold Exposure** – Cold temperatures lower your fight-or-flight response and strengthen the vagus nerve. Don't worry, you don't need to hop into an ice bath! Simply splashing your face with cold water in the morning is enough.
- **Diaphragmatic Breathing (Deep Breathing)** – Typically, people breathe on average about twelve times a minute. When our amygdala signals a threat, our breaths quicken, resulting in hyperventilation. If we breathe from our diaphragm and slow our breaths down to about six

breaths per minute, it activates the vagus nerve, which will tell your amygdala that there is no threat – thus reaching a state of calm and relaxation.

- **Singing, chanting, and gargling** – Your vagus nerve is connected to your vocal cords and throat muscles. Humming, singing, talking (calmly), and even chanting or gargling water triggers these muscles, stimulating your vagus nerve.

- **Probiotics** – A healthy gut leads to a healthy and focused mind. Have you ever felt run-down and fatigued but then ate something and felt ten times better? That's normal, but to increase your vagal tone, probiotics can strengthen your gut. Probiotics are found in

  - Yogurt
  - Sauerkraut
  - Kimchi
  - Pickles
  - Kefir

- **Massage** – Our bodies are surrounded and intertwined by nerve endings. Since the vagus nerve is the longest in our body, massaging certain parts of yourself stimulates the vagus nerve. You can ask a friend or hire a massage therapist to massage part of your feet, which will strengthen your vagal tone.

CHAPTER SUMMARY

In this chapter, we looked at;

- How anxiety is triggered by the amygdala searching for external threats.
- Why the amygdala initiates our fight-or-flight symptoms before the prefrontal-cortex even knows what's going on.
- How we can actively intercept this thought process
- Ways to help our brain and nervous system to combat our reactive anxiety

In the next chapter, we dive deeper into what's going on chemically in the brain and the impact of stress hormones on our bodies.

3

HORMONES AND STRESS

In this chapter we will look to understand:

- Stress hormones contributing to anxiety
- Actions to take to decrease stress hormones
- 'Feel good' hormones to decrease anxiety
- How we can increase 'happy' hormones

From the previous two chapters, we now understand a bit more about our brain and how it interprets threats from the external world. We know that the amygdala, which is always on high alert, can jump into action before our rational brain (PFC) has a chance to assess the situation.

Once the amygdala has decided there is an immediate threat, it sends out messages to prepare our bodies for action. We all know that sudden surge of energy we feel when confronted by something scary or dangerous. Almost instantaneously, the amygdala uses the nervous system to release three critical stress hormones; cortisol, adrenaline, and norepinephrine.

Many of the physical sensations we feel come from a surging release of these hormones to help fight the threat or run from it. But how does this happen? Well, the amygdala sends a distress signal to the hypothalamus (another part of the brain), which activates the parasympathetic nervous system. From there, signals are sent to the adrenal glands to release the three stress hormones; adrenaline (so that you can run faster or fight harder), cortisol (to curb non-essential functions to redirect energy to vital organs), and norepinephrine (to increase heart rate). It is essential to understand what these stress hormones do, how they make us feel and what we can do to manage them.

All three of these stress hormones are beneficial in our day-to-day lives. However, if they are released into the body too often and at high levels, they can have negative physical and psychological effects. Let me explain below:

CORTISOL

[1]We use cortisol throughout the day for good reason; for example, it is an important hormone that is released in the morning to wake us up. At its normal levels, cortisol regulates blood pressure and blood sugar levels and can even strengthen the heart muscles. Some studies have shown that higher-than-

normal levels of cortisol can help to improve memory recall and increase the pain threshold.

However, there is a danger that the amygdala would process the perceived threat too quickly and too often, and therefore our adrenal glands flood us with unnecessarily high levels of cortisol. Cortisol is a steroid hormone and gives us a heightened focus to concentrate on the stressful situation or impending threat. It is what gives us that feeling of being 'pumped'! It increases sugar levels in the bloodstream to give us an immediate energy source and takes any temporarily-stored sugar for us to use immediately. Cortisol also suppresses bodily processes that aren't essential, for example, our digestive system. This is one of the reasons why we feel nauseous and lose our appetites when we are stressed.

[2]The more we stew and focus on our lives' stressors, the more our adrenal glands will produce cortisol, causing the amygdala to produce unwanted flight-or-fight responses. It is essential to get a hold of our stress response system and engage in calming activities so that our bodies can produce balanced levels of cortisol. As mentioned, normal cortisol levels help keep our blood pressure, sugar, and immune systems balanced. However, too much stress will release a continuous amount of cortisol into our bodies. Not only will this trigger our amygdala, the excess cortisol will leave us with long-term health issues such as:

- Decreased libido
- Diabetes

- Heightened blood pressure
- Weakened immune system
- Acne
- Weight gain or loss

ADRENALINE

[3]As well as cortisol, our adrenal glands release adrenaline. It is the adrenaline that increases our heart rate and pumps our blood harder and faster, ready for swift action. It increases our heart rate and blood pressure and causes us to breathe more rapidly. The air passages in the lungs expand to take in as much oxygen as possible. This extra oxygen tells the brain to become even more alert and heighten all of our senses. I want to reiterate that all of this happens almost instantaneously, which is why we jump and squeal when somebody surprises us. Our PFC hasn't had time to process what is happening, and so the amygdala has gone into flight-or-fight mode within seconds.

[4]The more stress you have in your life, the more your adrenal glands will produce adrenaline. When this happens, you may end up with overactive adrenal glands, which will release too much adrenaline and norepinephrine too many times. Basically, more stress adds to constant heightened awareness, which leads to an overload of anxiety, which is essentially a constant flow of adrenaline rush. This high frequency of adrenaline surges can damage blood vessels over

time, increase anxiety, create insomnia, and result in headaches and a lowered immune system.

Both of these stress hormones (cortisol and adrenaline) are vital for us daily. From getting us up in the morning to catching the bus. We don't want to stop producing stress hormones, but it is crucial to understand their part in our physical sensations of anxiety.

NOREPINEPHRINE

Adrenaline and norepinephrine are very similar hormones that get released into our bloodstreams. However, the main difference is that norepinephrine is a constant flow of hormones released at low levels to feel alert, focused, and attentive in our daily lives. On the other hand, adrenaline only gets released in a larger dose when a supposed threat is at hand. Norepinephrine is responsible for shifting blood flow to other regions in our bodies that need it. For example, if you have ever stubbed your toe or sprained your ankle and you need to elevate it, norepinephrine sends blood to that part of your body as part of the healing process.

Although you might think, 'Why do I need adrenaline if I have norepinephrine?' or vice versa, they are both important. Think of norepinephrine as a backup supply of adrenaline and vice versa. Once your adrenaline levels have dropped, you may feel tired, exhausted, and weak. Well, this is where epinephrine gives your body the strength to continue after a stressful episode or anxiety attack.

Actions to Take:

There are a few ways to manage and even reduce the number of stress hormones our adrenal glands produce.

- **Physical activity**

To keep our stress hormones at a manageable level, it is essential to understand that taking regular exercise not only reduces our feelings of stress but also relieves muscle tension, which induces calm. Although intense exercise initially increases cortisol, studies have found that interestingly, cortisol levels significantly decrease at night following intense exercise during the day. Meaning if you can find the energy for a strenuous workout throughout the day, you will feel much more relaxed and calm at night.

- **Sleep**

[5]An episode of insomnia causes significantly higher levels of cortisol for up to twenty-four hours. Cortisol is produced by the hypothalamic-pituitary-adrenal **(HPA)** axis. When we are sleeping, our minds go through three stages. The first stage consists of drifting into sleep. Second, our core temperature drops, allowing our brainwaves to become slower. The third is known as the 'slow-wave sleep' which means our brainwaves, heart rate, and breathing are at their lowest points. Finally, our bodies become relaxed enough that we fall into REM (rapid eye movement)

sleep. This entire process happens within ninety minutes of laying down to rest. Having an overly active HPA can disrupt our sleep, which results in experiencing insomnia, interrupted sleep, or a generally shortened period of time when we are resting. When our HPA is overactive, it produces significant amounts of cortisol, which, as you have learned, is your stress response. When we do not get enough sleep through the night or not at all, we feel dazed, unfocused, and restless. During the day, our melatonin levels drop, which makes our brains think that we need to become focused and alert. So, the HPA releases high levels of cortisol into our bodies to help us stay focused and alert. No wonder we can't sleep at night. According to the American Institute of Stress, when we get a full rested night's worth of sleep, our bodies are less likely to feel on edge or tense the next day.

In chapter five, we will look at practical, implementable ways to improve our exercise routines and sleep patterns.

- **Aromatherapy**

Soothing scents are natural ways to reduce our stress hormone levels and increase relaxation in our lives so that we are better equipped to handle a stressful event when it happens (rather than freaking out). Some anxiety-reducing scents include:

- Lavender
- Bergamont

- Chamomile
- Sandalwood
- Orange Blossom
- Frankincense

- **Balanced diet**

Try creating a diet schedule. What will you have for breakfast, lunch, and dinner? But make sure to leave room for healthy snacks in-between. A good rule of thumb is to make sure you keep a nutrition bar on you when you are planning to go out. Try supplementation. A few natural supplements that you can take at any time every day to lower your stress hormones include:

- Lemon Balm
- Omega-3 fatty Acids
- Ashwagandha
- Green tea (L-Theanine)
- Valerian root

BRAIN COMMUNICATION SYSTEM & NEUROTRANSMITTERS

The brain is the mothership and the control center, and so it needs a way to communicate. It does this using neurons and neurotransmitters.

Neurons are the nerve cells that receive messages from our surroundings and send commands to other parts of the body to respond. There are about eighty billion neurons in the brain whose sole purpose is to communicate with one another to interpret and translate the world around us. Every thought, feeling, emotion, and memory you have ever had is because of these neurons communicating with one another. However, these neurons can't touch one another to pass on their messages; there is always a gap between them. This gap is called a synapse. To communicate across this gap, neurons 'throw' their messages to one another using chemicals called neurotransmitters.

These neurotransmitters carry the message from one neuron to another and electrically charge that neuron to pass the message on and cause us to take action. It is hard to over-estimate the importance of these neurotransmitters and the messages they carry. Sometimes they don't carry enough charge to fire up the next neuron, and the messaging system stops. Sometimes they carry too much, and the 'leftovers' are sucked back up by the neuron that sent the message.

There are many neurotransmitters the brain uses, but the ones we are really interested in regarding anxiety are dopamine and serotonin.

DOPAMINE

Dopamine is often called the 'feel-good' chemical as it drives us to pursue activities that give us joy or help us achieve our goals. When dopamine is released in large amounts, it creates feelings of pleasure and motivates us to repeat a specific behavior. In contrast, low levels of dopamine are linked to reduced motivation and decreased enthusiasm for things that most people enjoy. Dopamine is a critical component in our reward system that moves us to action in achieving our goals. It is the reward we get for completing tasks we strive for or consuming things we crave. Dopamine gives us feelings of desire and curiosity, as well as the motivation to satisfy them. It does this by creating reward circuits in the brain so that we will repeat the behavior. The circuit logs an activity as intensely pleasurable and vital, to tell the brain to repeat the behavior again and again.

This would be great if we could create these circuits attached only to positive behaviors such as exercise. Still, all too often, dopamine loops are created from more sedentary activities, like Instagram scrolling or Netflix binging.

Recently, neuroscientists have shown that dopamine isn't just released as a reward for achieving a behavior. It also rewards the effort process. As you pass milestones to a goal, you also release dopamine to encourage and motivate you on your journey. This is really exciting because we can encourage our brains to release dopamine more regularly to help us combat our anxious brain and motivate us to behave in ways that reduce anxiety.

HOW TO INCREASE DOPAMINE LEVELS

[6]Having clear goals and milestones are critical in increasing our dopamine levels. These goals do not have to be climbing Mount Everest, by the way! An example of one of my previous goals is below:

Goal – I will run 3k within five weeks.
Week 1 – Milestone 1 – I will run twice this week for 1k
Week 2 – Milestone 2 – I will run twice this week for 1.5k
Week 3 – Milestone 3 – I will run three times this week for 2k
Week 4 – Milestone 4 – I will run twice this week for 2.5k
Week 5 – Milestone 5 – I will run 3k

As the weeks pass and you see achievements towards your goal, your dopamine levels increase. This increase occurs not only from achieving the milestones you set, but also as a result of *anticipating* achieving the next milestone! The goal itself doesn't matter too much as long as it's a stretch goal for you, something that can be broken down to measurable milestones and something you want to achieve. It should be something positive, too, and not related to pursuing negative behavior. We will go into goal-setting more in chapter seven.

You can also increase dopamine levels through your diet. Foods rich in tyrosine are said to increase the release of dopamine. These foods include cheese, meats, fish, dairy, soy, seeds, nuts, beans, and lentils. As with any dietary advice, try to avoid processed foods, high-fats, sugar, and caffeine. But you knew that would be in here somewhere. Other dopamine-increasing foods include:

- Probiotics (you can find a list back in chapter 2)
- Velvet beans (Mucuna pruriens)
- Almonds
- Fresh fruit (from the produce section)
- Green vegetables (leafy greens, broccoli, green peppers)
- Green tea (L-theanine)

Exercise and good sleep habits are also critical as they fuel dopamine production – more on sleep and exercise in chapter five. However, anything you can think of that makes you happy, more confident, or helps you achieve something increases your dopamine levels.

SEROTONIN

Serotonin cannot cross the blood-brain barrier, so any serotonin used inside the brain must be produced inside the brain. Serotonin is most commonly believed to be a neurotransmitter, although some consider it to be a hormone. It is produced in the intestines and the brain. It is also present in the blood platelets and the central nervous system (CNS).

Serotonin's effects in the brain could be considered its 'starring role' in the body. As it helps regulate our moods, serotonin is often called the body's natural 'feel-good' chemical. Serotonin's influence on mood makes it one of several brain chemicals that are integral to our overall sense of well-being.

The neurotransmitter's effect on mood is also why it's often a target of medications that are used to treat depression, anxiety, and other mood disorders as many are closely linked to low levels of serotonin.

HOW TO INCREASE SEROTONIN

[7]Vitamin B is an excellent place to start looking to increase serotonin. B vitamins help turn tryptophan and amino acid from proteins into serotonin. No wonder people feel happy and calm after eating turkey at Christmas! Other things that help increase serotonin levels are:[8]

- Sunlight or Vitamin C during winter months
- Light lamp
- Spending time in nature or outside
- Exercise
- Reminiscing on happy memories
- Achieving a goal

CHAPTER SUMMARY

We covered a lot in this chapter relating to;

- The impact hormones have on our anxiety and how we can use them to our advantage.
- Acknowledging when our stress hormones are working against us
- How to increase those all important 'feel good' hormones

4

SELF-TALK AND JOURNALING

In this chapter we will look at ways to build resilience to anxiety through:

- Positive self-talk and how it can be used
- Habits
- Thinking traps
- The benefits of journaling

To get anxiety under control, we must make conscious choices towards changing aspects of our lives to live without fear and anxiety. When we have lived with anxiety for so long, the things contributing to our anxiety disorder become habitual. For example, if we have long-term anxiety, we can get trapped into a mindset which dictates our behavior. Like we talked about in the last chapter, we may start avoiding situations that bring on anxiety, such as going out in public or talking to strangers. So, to make it simple; our thoughts contribute to our anxiety, which then contributes to our avoidance behavior, which also keeps anxiety along for the ride. We want to stop this pattern, so let's talk about two simple techniques that are incredibly powerful and effective.

POSITIVE SELF-TALK AND AFFIRMATIONS

[1]This is a conscious way of talking to yourself in a positive and supportive way. Our brains process approximately 40,000 thoughts a day, and according to the National Science Foundation, 80% of these are negative. These thoughts are often going on unnoticed to us in the background and repeated over and over throughout the day. It would be impossible to be aware of our every thought and challenge all the negative ones. However, we can interrupt the pattern by consciously inserting positive self-talk and affirmations.

Affirmations help soothe our anxious minds when we feel anxiety rising. It is one way to challenge our negative thoughts and anxiety thinking traps. Like anything that we want to achieve or change in our lives, we need to make it a habit and repeat it daily to master it. Essentially, once we actively repeat affirmations every day, over time, we will become more resilient to stressful situations. That way, positive self-talk becomes proactive rather than counteractive during a full-blown anxiety attack. The trick is to calm down before the anxiety hits, which is what affirmations are used for. So, let's take a more in-depth look:

HOW TO USE AFFIRMATIONS

Using affirmations to ease anxiety is as easy as breathing. When you feel anxiety rising, sit down, close your eyes, and take a deep breath. Then quietly speak to yourself and use positive and truthful statements such as:

- I am okay. This is only anxiety, and it will pass.
- I know that my feelings are just feelings and I am completely safe.
- My amygdala is reacting to something it perceives as threatening right now. There is no threat. I am safe.
- I am safe. I am strong. I am calm and I am relaxing.
- I acknowledge my anxiety. I also acknowledge it will pass.

Do you see how each affirmation centers your attention away from your feelings and ends with a positive statement of truth? This is how affirmations are used. You can repeat them as many times as you would like until you feel calmer and move onto another coping mechanism. The tone of voice in your mind should be as calm and soothing as you can manage.

Affirmations activate the brain systems associated with reward (dopamine) and how the brain makes future predictions. Therefore, positive self-talk helps improve our resilience to stress, which creates a more positive outlook for our future. This is essentially how we create habits.

HABITS

[2]Habits are created in four steps. First, we have a cue, then a craving, next is the response to the craving, and then a reward that solidifies the habit. Once this has been repeated over time, the habit becomes mastered, and now we're doing it without question. For example, brushing your teeth. The cue is imagining or having the picture of a toothbrush pop in your head. The craving is the taste of mint or the smell of freshness on your breath. The response is brushing your teeth, and the reward is fulfilling your craving.

Let's take a closer look:

The cue is the trigger for the craving you need satisfied. Practically, the brain sees cues everywhere around us and is always working on building habits and routines because it relies mostly on a structure. Hence, anxiety becomes an anxiety disorder because we're triggered (cue), then automatically, the amygdala is searching for the craving to fulfill the trigger. Once the craving becomes fulfilled (such as avoidance behavior), our anxiety dissipates by using positive affirmations or meditation (our response to our trigger and craving). Finally, the reward is no feelings of anxiety. This creates new neural connections in your brain to say, 'Hey, let's do that again.' So, essentially you just taught your brain to use your cravings to calm anxiety by using a coping mechanism to reduce, and then your reward is no feelings of fear or concern.

Now that is a healthy way of dealing with anxiety, but our anxiety gets out of control most of the time because we have already created an unhealthy habit surrounding how we deal with our panic. For example, we see a rope on the floor (cue/trigger), but our minds see it as a snake 'OMG, it's a snake,' (amygdala working overtime, negative thinking trap sets in). We run away and hide (craving to reduce the fear and anxiety we feel), then once we are away from the rope, our symptoms start to dissipate (the response activated from fulfilling your craving). Once the anxiety symptoms go away entirely, we have achieved our reward (what we wanted from the experience.) You have now just taught your brain to run away and avoid things to get your reward.

Other examples of the habit loop are:

- The phone vibrates or makes a sound (cue). We become curious to know why (craving). We grab our phone to check it out (response). The craving disappears because we fulfilled the curiosity for why the phone made a sound (reward).
- We smell enticing food (cue). We now crave whatever we smelled (craving). We detour to where we smell the food or buy the ingredients, and eat it

(response). We satisfy our craving by eating the entire meal (reward).

- We see someone attractive (cue). We feel the need to talk to them or plan a date (craving). We walk up to them and start a conversation that may or may not lead to a date (response). We fulfilled the need to start a conversation with the attractive person and got your date (reward).

[3] As you can see, habits are everywhere. They are everything we do, from waking up in the morning to sleeping at night. Habits can help with your anxiety if you start to understand your habit's cue, craving, response, and reward system. From here onwards, please take a look into your anxiety triggers, and find out what you currently do to solve it or reduce it to get your reward. Once we do this, we can start changing our behavior the next time (and the next time) our anxiety kicks in. We can replace our anxiety cravings by becoming curious to know what our craving is when an attack occurs. Since most of the time, all we want is to calm down, find a calming and healthy option to satisfy your craving, and over time, you will get the reward you desire in the end. We all know the end goal (reward) is to not let our fear and panic control our lives.

Now that you understand a little more about how habits work, we can focus on how to input positive affirmations into our daily routine to set off our reward (dopamine) system and ultimately beat anxiety. Below are some of my favorite affirmations that I use regularly.

- 'May I be happy, may I be safe, may I be healthy, may I be at peace.'
- 'I breathe in calm and breathe out tension.'
- 'I am living a calm and compassionate life.'
- 'This feeling is anxiety, and I will be extra gentle with myself until it passes.'
- 'Anxiety isn't dangerous. I'm just uncomfortable, and it will pass.'

I repeat one of these statements at least five times in a row. I usually like to say them to myself while I am outside walking, as that is when I am less distracted. But you can do them anywhere at any time. Try them and see how they feel.

Although you can use these affirmations at any given time, try them out when you are having an anxiety attack as your first attempt to calm yourself. You will see that not only will you feel calmer, you will also feel more equipped to assess and identify why the anxiety started – remember *chapter two* under *the prefrontal cortex?*

Affirmations are not just an anxiety-calming technique but also a strategy that upbeat and high-energy people use in their everyday lives. All it takes is a little practice making something this easy a habit to change your mindset from 'Ahh! Run!' to 'Step aside, anxiety, I have got this.'

Thinking (anxiety) traps are what happens with our

thoughts when our amygdalas perceive a threat or some form of danger. Basically, these traps make us believe the lies we tell ourselves and keep us in a pattern of fear and anxiety. Over time, these traps keep us inside our heads, altering our ability to think rationally which becomes our first response to just about everything.

THINKING TRAPS (ANXIETY TRAPS)

> 'OMG, my heart is racing. I am experiencing a
>   heart attack.'
> 'She looked at me wrong. She must not
>   like me.'
> 'Well, I am bad at this, so I guess I am bad at
>   everything.'
> 'I was late for my appointment. I can never do
>   anything right.'

[4]Sound familiar? Have you had at least one of these thoughts before? Well, these are thinking traps. It's a state of mind where our thoughts say something, and we automatically believe it. If we thought it, it must be true, right? Wrong! The truth is, a thought is just a thought. That's all it is. A feeling is just a feeling. The only reason we believe in our thoughts and feelings so deeply is that we genuinely believe the misinformation our brains are trying to tell us. It's a matter of perception. Look at it this way, if your best friend calls to

tell you that your current boyfriend or girlfriend is spreading lies about you, are you going to believe it right away, or would you look into it first? Your rational mind would want to look into it first, but your emotional mind would believe your best friend because, well, they are your best friend and would never lie to you. That's how anxiety or thinking traps work. Our best friend (Anxiety) is telling us one thing, and our emotional mind (amygdala) believes it off the bat without looking into it with our rational mind (prefrontal cortex).

Here are 10 of the most common Thinking Traps:

Thinking Trap	What's Happening?	Example
Black and White/ All or Nothing	We only see one side or the other. There is no grey matter in between	Failed once or got one thing wrong. 'I am obviously too dumb, so why try it ever again?'
Catastrophizing	The worst thing will happen, no matter what, even if it seems highly unlikely	The power goes out. 'We are going to live in darkness forever, now I am going to starve, and I won't be able to socialize with anyone ever again.'
Overestimating	An exaggerated likelihood that something bad is already happening	Plant or broom falls on the floor without a logical explanation. 'Omg, we are having an earthquake right now!'
Telling the Future	Thinking you know the future	'I failed my class, so that means I am going to fail every other class.'
Overgeneralizing	Using the words always or never (similar to black and white thinking)	'I am always late. I will never be on time,' or 'I have always embarrassed myself. I will never get a date.'
Mind-reading	Thinking you know what others are thinking about you	'I know she thinks little of me.' Or, 'I know they are talking about me.'
Negative Views	Nothing is ever positive. Everything you see is negative, no matter what	'I got one question wrong on my test, so I am a failure' even though you passed.
Personalization	You are always the cause, even if you're not	'My partner is mad, it's because of me.'
Should and Shouldn't	Overthinking about what had happened and what you could have done differently to change things	'I should have spoken up' or 'I shouldn't have looked their way.'
Emotional Reasoning	You think something, so it must be true	'I think I look bad, so I must look horrible.'

JOURNALING

[5]When we put our thoughts into writing, we can get out what we have been holding onto and then take a step back and read through what we wrote. For me, journaling my thoughts and continuously working through my anxiety (rather than against it) made me learn patience and compassion for myself. This helps us in two ways.

Firstly, we get our thoughts out – even if they are unorganized and unplanned. Pick up a blank page and start writing whatever comes to your mind because, honestly, it's only for our eyes to read, so why do we need to make it look pretty? If we write when we're upset, angry, or anxious, we are so focused on writing what's on our minds that we end up writing a full page, and then afterward, it's as if there has been a weight lifted from our shoulders.

Secondly, when you go over and re-read your entry, you may notice that some things aren't as big as you were previously blowing them up. If you keep a weekly journal, you can go back and re-read at any time. You will start to see a pattern of your emotional behavior, allowing you to become self-aware and resolve the issue.

- **Prevents negative thoughts and thinking traps**

Some journal entries, you don't even need to keep. For example, if you wrote something so debilitating and stressful that you have no idea how to relieve tension from it, you can throw it away or burn it (following safety precautions, either on an established fire or over a sink). A study from Psychological Science Journal in 2011 noted that you could effectively clear your mind by doing so. The study tested high-school students in Spain. The research consisted of the students writing down their body image beliefs and then being asked to throw it away afterward. The results showed that the students who followed through with the experiment didn't show body image thoughts later in life. That said, journaling can be a healthy release if you need to get those pesky negative thoughts out of your head and then throw the entry away or burn it.

- **Enhances problem-solving skills**

When we think about our anxiety, and we understand that it has become a habit, it starts to control our lives because of our behavior connected to our routines. Problem-solving skills are about understanding how to identify the problem and then coming up with a logical explanation as to why it happened so that we can solve the related issue. When we write our problems down, we can visualize them better and start writing a structured plan to solve them. When you read what you have written at a later date, you will see if what you wrote in the current moment is similar to your previous entries. In doing so, you can recognize patterns, which will help you solve the current problems you're experiencing.

- **Significantly reduces stress**

By understanding our habits brought on by anxiety, our tolerance of stress and the ability to manage our heightened emotions will dramatically increase. If we can take a step back and realize that we felt one hundred times better by the end of our journal entry, that overall will make us feel more accomplished. It will also set us up to reduce stress during stressful events because when we notice our patterns, we will notice it's like any other time and won't fear it anymore.

- **Improves Physical Health**

The American Medical Association journal conducted a study about participants with chronic illnesses who journaled their thoughts and stressful life events. The result of the experiment was that out of the 112 patients, those who wrote in a journal experienced fewer physical symptoms than the ones who didn't journal at all. After four months, the group showed a fifty percent improvement rate with their physical ailments.

- **Improves Self-Awareness**

When we write our thoughts and feelings down, we become more aware of them when we experience them first-hand. When we become self-aware, we can make instant conscious reactions to the anxiety and panic we feel at that moment. Self-awareness also helps with other things in life, including healthy relationships, improvement at work and school, and accomplishing goals and dreams in our personal lives.

So, if journaling is so positive, how do we do it? Here are some different types of journaling you can try:

Gratitude Journal

A gratitude journal is a journal where we write down every day what we are grateful for at the time. Whether this is a whole list of things, or just a few things, or the same things, it's the process of writing down what we're thankful for that helps our brains release stress. By keeping a gratitude journal, we can look back on the things we enjoy and appreciate when we feel depressed or angry. Essentially, writing and reading these back will create a positive environment, which will help us keep a positive perspective on the world. Gratitude journals are helpful because as we write down what we are thankful for, we realize that there is more positivity in our lives than we thought. It helps us to take a step back from cynicism and anger while also uplifting our overall attitudes, and to envision bigger and brighter future.

Diary

Diaries are recommended to those who need a regular or as-needed emotional release. These journals help us process our thoughts and emotions and release the anxiety and anger rather than bottling it up and releasing it on someone else. A Diary is also used for writing positive experiences so that we can look back and remember, 'that was a good day'. Ultimately, this will keep us happier and increase our levels of serotonin and dopamine hormones.

Planner

A planner is a type of journal where we write down our to-dos. This journal helps us stay organized and productive. If we are more productive, we're more focused and confident. Confidence boosts our moods and keeps our minds uncluttered, which relieves stress and anxiety symptoms. Make your planner special by adding stickers, highlights, sticky notes, photos, and memories. Think of it as your blog that shows you your accomplishments and helps you stay motivated to complete the other things on your bullet list.

CHAPTER SUMMARY

As we grow to understand our anxiety, we start to understand how to calm our anxiety before it begins. We learn how to do this through our state of mind. If we are negative, we are always going to see negativity around us. Positive affirmations are one thing we can use to reduce anxious symptoms and become more resilient when a stressful event happens in the present moment. However, much like anything else, it takes practice and commitment to make these healthy changes in our lives to become resilient and strong against our fears, which is why habits are set in place.

Try to introduce positive, new habits such as:

- Daily affirmations
- Recognise your thinking traps and challenge them
- Daily gratitude journal
- Feelings diary

5

WHY EXERCISE AND SLEEP SHOULD BE TOP OF OUR TO-DO LISTS

I know you know this already. We only have to do a quick Google search for anxiety advice, and it immediately suggests regular exercise and good sleeping patterns for reducing anxiety. But I also know that when we feel anxious, committing to exercise and getting eight hours of sleep isn't always possible. So, if we know exercise and sleep are critical for reducing anxiety, how can we make them achievable when we need them the most?

In this chapter, we will look at:

- The benefits of exercise
- What counts as exercise
- The benefits of regular, sufficient sleep
- How to sleep better

THE BENEFITS OF EXERCISE

[1]Firstly, let's remind ourselves why exercise is so beneficial for calming our anxious brains.

- **Decreases stress hormones. Increases 'feel good' hormones.** As we discussed previously, when we are anxious, cortisol and adrenaline work together to induce the unpleasant anxiety symptoms. This, in turn, causes us to worry about the severity of these symptoms ('What if this is not anxiety?' 'What if there is something wrong?'). Ruminating about our feelings and sensations causes significant stress, which builds tension, causing even more physical symptoms. The vicious cycle then repeats, causing us to become a victim to our thinking traps. Exercise breaks this cycle because it releases anti-anxiety hormones and neurochemicals like endorphins, serotonin, and Gamma-aminobutyric Acid (GABA). All of which improve feelings of well-being and build resilience.
- **Physical activity distracts us from negative thoughts and emotions.** Physical activity can distract the brain from overly focusing on negative thoughts and redirect its focus. Exercise provides an opportunity for the prefrontal cortex to take the lead and the amygdala to step back. In doing so, the brain has time to focus on motivation,

memories, and problem-solving. Essentially, when we exercise, we have no time to focus on all the pessimistic stuff that tries to enter our world and instead allow rational PFC to work through our thoughts.

- **Exercise can be a good source of social support.** Our human instinct for survival is to be around other people and use them for support and advice. Our social connections and learning from one another have thrust our evolution forward at such speed. Without regular social interaction with people with shared beliefs and goals, we can isolate, which is a huge contributor to depression and anxiety. However, when we feel depressed or anxious, it is incredibly hard to put ourselves into social situations. By exercising with someone or in a group, we benefit from social support and connection without the pressure of being 'sociable'. So whether you join an exercise class or you play softball in a league, grab an exercise buddy and get a double-dose of stress relief.

- **Exercise provides a buffer against stress**. Physical activity may be linked to lower physiological reactivity toward stress. Simply put, those who get more exercise may become less affected by the stress they face. So, in addition to all the other benefits, exercise may supply some resilience to stressful situations in your life. This is because the higher the dose of endorphins and feel-good hormones that enter your system, the less often your anxiety-reacting hormones will be released, resulting in a less anxiety-filled life.

[2]NOW LET'S LOOK AT HOW WE CAN GET EXERCISE IN OUR life when our anxious brains don't want us to.

- **Go outside!**

No matter what the weather, get outside for at least twenty minutes daily. Initially, it doesn't matter what you are doing outside; just being in the fresh air and the sense of moving forward will help. Remember, anxiety symptoms are trying to get you to move away from danger, and so by moving, even at a walk, your brain will recognize you are taking action and begin to calm the amygdala and give the PFC a chance. When I am particularly anxious, I find running spurts and then walking are incredibly helpful. You don't need a gym kit or even trainers. Just run for ten seconds, then walk for three minutes, then run for ten more seconds and walk for another three minutes, and so on. It not only gives your brain something to concentrate on, but it also gets rid of some of the excess norepinephrine we don't need.

- **At home**

If you really can't get outside because of childcare or other commitments, then you can do things at home. Start by running on the spot for twenty seconds and then walk on the spot for three minutes and repeat three more times. Again, this will give your brain something to focus on and calm the amygdala. Try some yoga poses if you can. I know this is hard when we are anxious because everything feels too heightened to stay in one pose for long periods. However, it is said that yoga is one of the best exercises to train our brains to be less anxious. This is because, during yoga, we learn deeper concentration through breathing techniques. Our minds are too focused on the workout itself to become anxious about anything else, and yoga teaches us mantra statements which we will discuss a little later. Still unsure? Trying for ten minutes is enough. There are plenty of Youtube resources for beginner yoga, but I particularly like *Yoga with Adriene*. Just put it on and do it when you can! I promise you will be glad you did, even after only ten minutes.

- **Classes**

If you are lucky enough to have a gym membership and feel you have the motivation to go, that is awesome! Interacting with strangers, bonding over a shared experience and goal can be immensely uplifting. But if that isn't something you feel you can do yet, then don't worry. That can be something to aim for in the future. Let's make it one of your long-term goals! There are all types of classes, from yoga to Tae-Kwon-Do (which is a great workout, by the way), to personal fitness, etc... Pick something you think you would be interested in, and choose a date. It's okay if you happen to chicken out the first few times; anxiety can do this to many of us. However, keep trying so that you don't teach your brain that it's okay to give up. You can try to search for fitness classes on Youtube or buy workout disks from a store. You can do this from the comfort of your own home while watching others take the class with you on your TV. Although this isn't something that should take over social workouts, it's the first step towards your goal.

While it's important to know that we can at least decrease our anxiety through exercise, and the above information gives us some great options, the real obstacle can often be those pesky thoughts that might get in the way before we even start. You know what I mean – those excuses that we come up with that tell ourselves, 'I don't have time right now'. Then it never gets done. Or 'I will get to this later,' and we become distracted or anxious, and that's what we spend our time focusing on. No worries, just like any new habit you are hopeful to start, you can train your brain to become committed and motivated. Don't give up. Here are some ways to stay on track when you're struggling.

STICKING WITH IT

Doing something new always takes work and overcoming the obstacles we run into, such as excuses or anxiety. Knowing the benefits of exercise and how it significantly decreases feelings of anxiety is our motivation. However, when it comes right down to exercising, we must take steps to do so. It's almost impossible to get up one day and run a 10k when we haven't built up our lung resilience to do so. Or, there is the other possibility where we are doing so great for a week straight – getting up every day and doing yoga, or going for a light jog, or just doing simple stretches at home along with some sit-ups and spot-running. But then after about a week, we start exercising only four times a week, then two, and eventually none. So, how do we keep the momentum going to keep exercising as a life change – doing it every day?

- **Get rid of those excuses. Ignore your thinking traps**

Excuses like 'I hate exercise' or 'I'm too tired today' or 'I'm not an athlete' are all or nothing thinking. Your first goal is to challenge these thoughts. I suggest creating a workout journal or a thought journal. When your mind goes, 'I'm too tired,' write that down but then write a response saying something like, 'I may be tired, but that's because my anxiety is trying to stop me from getting better. If I start slow, I will feel better, which will decrease my anxiety symptoms'. When your mind says, 'I hate exercising,' challenge it by saying, 'exercise is good for me, and it will help me decrease my anxiety. What's worse, having panic attacks or going for a walk?'

- **Create a starter routine**

Firstly, make a list of all the workouts that sound the best to you, and start with the one you want to try. Before doing it, start with a warm-up, which could be stretching, jogging on the spot, or listening to your favorite pumped-up music. Get yourself in the mood and start your first week just doing light exercises like warm-ups and cool-downs. That way, you can get a feel for what feels right to you, and during the second week, add something after your warm-up. This could be stretching, then going outside for a brisk jog, and then your cool-down period could be walking all the way home, or even simply walking up and down the stairs several times.

- **Choose a workout buddy**.

Do you have a friend that suffers from anxiety too? Or maybe you know someone positive, upbeat, and energetic? Pick a friend and ask them if they want to be your workout buddy. Not only will this help you get out of your comfort zone in small doses, it will also help you become motivated for the days you don't feel like exercising. Or if your friend feels low and comes up with their excuses, you can call them and motivate them. Together, you can find a flow that works and your new habit forms into a daily exercise routine.

- **Keep what you love**

Remember that exercise list? After about four weeks of slowly working up to a daily exercise routine, you should know what works for you and what doesn't. Once you know that, you can choose what you love the most from your list and continue with this until you are ready to learn and experience more.

- **Reward yourself**

In the previous chapter, I explained what habits were and talked about the habit loop. There is always a reward system that solidifies your craving from the habit loop, making it an enforced habit. It's the same thing with exercise. Before you start your daily workout routine, make sure you have a plan in place to reward yourself after fulfilling your daily goal. This could be treating yourself to a food you love, getting a massage, or using up the entire hot water tank in your home for a much-needed relaxing shower.

One of the best things about exercise is it burns adrenaline, which helps relaxation and, in turn, aids sleep. When we feel restless or wide awake at night, it could stem from the very fact that we aren't active enough during the day.

SLEEP

[3]Sleep has always been my nemesis. I spent years chasing that elusive eight hours. I would be exhausted all day, and then as soon as I went to bed, I would be ultra alert and awake. I would lie there and become more awake as the night went on. My mind would repeat, 'Just go to sleep' but I would feel hot, nauseous, fidgety, and desperate. It became a disastrous pattern of not sleeping because I was anxious, followed by anxiety about not sleeping and, therefore, not sleeping. The world is an extraordinary place when you don't sleep. It is impossible to hold concentration, rationalize thoughts, let alone have the energy to exercise.

I found the less I slept, the more anxious I became about not sleeping, and then the anxiety fed on this feeling in a perfect circle of worry. Firstly, it is essential to remember that sleep eludes most people at some time, whether because of stress, stimulants, hormones, or simply the 'Sunday night' feeling. It is not unusual, and it is not dangerous. It is annoying and frustrating and can mess up your day, but that's it! Also, you may be adamant you didn't sleep a wink...when in reality, you probably did drift off for a few minutes here and there.

For me, I know that sleep is a crucial anxiety trigger, and I know it has to be a priority, as much as diet and exercise. These are a few of the tactics I use to hack my brain when it doesn't switch off:

- **Don't try to sleep!**

If I know I am very anxious and too anxious to sleep, I don't try. Ideally, I go to bed with a book and ask my other half to sleep on the sofa just for a night, so I don't keep him awake too!

- **Journal**

Then with a low light on, I write down anything in my head, not necessarily worries, but a brain dump of everything swirling around in my mind. I tell myself, 'I probably won't sleep tonight, and that's okay'. It's no big deal, just mildly annoying. When we don't put pressure on ourselves to fall asleep, our brains focus on other things, letting sleep happen naturally. Before you know it, it's lights out.

- **Read a book**

Next, I read and let my mind wander. I usually find I fall asleep with my book on my face at some point. I don't get eight hours of sleep, but I do get a few hours, which is enough to reassure me for the day ahead.

- **Commit to a sleep plan**

[4]Routine is the key to sleep. The brain likes a healthy sleep pattern, so it knows when to release melatonin (the hormone

to make you sleepy) and when to wake us up. So let's help it out and give it a routine, so it knows what to expect. Much like forming new habits, the exact times can be amended depending on your personal home situation but the following works for me:

- No caffeine after 15.00
- No screens, including TV thirty minutes before bed
- Go to bed at eleven at night and read for thirty minutes
- Light off no later than midnight
- Get up every day no later than eight in the morning

Try out your nightly schedule, which often can include things like meditation, listening to lulling music, or opening the window. The goal is to ensure that your brain isn't distracted or busy at least an hour before you intend to get some shut-eye. This means no TV, no electronics, and no planning for your future or even tomorrow. When your body is relaxed and comfortable, your mind will follow suit, which will lead to an increase in melatonin, ultimately leaving your body and mind enough time to say, 'Hey, I am tired, let's go to sleep now'.

Life sometimes makes sleep plans impossible, but I find as long as I stick to this 80% of the time, I very rarely have problems sleeping now.

. . .

[5]SOME READERS MAY BE LOOKING AT THIS RIGHT NOW and thinking, 'I have literally tried everything, and this still doesn't work for me'. Fortunately, there are more things we can try. Rather than prescribed sleep aids, there are natural sleep-inducing natural supplements that are widely known to help:

Vitamins

- Vitamin C
- Iron
- Magnesium
- Vitamin B12
- Tryptophan
- Melatonin
- Vitamin D
- Calcium

Supplements

- Lavender scented items
- GABA supplements
- Valerian Root
- CBD oil
- Kava Kava
- Chamomile
- 5-HTP

- Passionflower

Essential Oils (Aromatherapy)

- Lavender
- Peppermint
- Sandalwood
- Bergamont
- Sweet Marjoram
- Chamomile
- Vanilla
- Valarian
- Frankincense

I want to take a moment to stress that I am not a doctor, but the things I previously mentioned are based on my personal experiences and research. The methods I explain throughout this book have been tried, tested, and implemented by me and others I know and have met. It's one thing to research something, and another to put the research into practice. I have tried, practiced, and watched as others cure and cope with their anxiety through the methods I talk about in this book. Part of changing and rebuilding our lives is being persistent as we try to live with less anxiety. With the supplements I mentioned, it's best not to try all of them at once, but talk to your family practitioner and ask them about the supplements and vitamins you would like to try to calm your anxiety naturally. And, of course, which are best to take together and which to take as needed. The vitamins act differently, and you will need to take these during the day for a couple of months for your long-term goal of achieving REM sleep.

CHAPTER SUMMARY

Sleep and exercise go hand-in-hand when it comes to reducing the severity of our daily anxious symptoms. In this chapter, we have covered:

- The benefits of exercise
- How to stick with and make exercise a daily habit
- The importance of sleep and what works for me personally
- Other things you can try to get some shut-eye
- Speak with your doctor first before taking any supplements or vitamins together

6

BREATHING – IN THE MOMENT AND OUT OF THE MOMENT

This chapter will introduce breathing techniques for anxiety and specifically:

- The difference between thoracic and diaphragmatic breathing.
- What 'in the moment' breathing is.
- What 'out of the moment' breathing is
- Meditation exercises and techniques

A whole chapter based on breathing may seem a little extreme; however, I have found that breathing exercises are one of the most effective ways of combating anxiety and panic attacks. Although breathing for anxiety will take some practice, it will help to understand why it works. Therefore in this chapter, I want to cover why breathing exercises work and give some examples that you can try.

Breathing is something we take for granted because we do it all the time without thinking. We would assume our bodies know how to breathe effectively as they've had all of our lives to practice! Breathing is part of our autonomic system, which means it happens involuntarily without us having to think or intervene. Just like our heartbeat and digestion, breathing is happening all the time subconsciously. However, breathing is the only autonomic system we have that we can also actively control. When we breathe slowly, powerfully, and with concentration, it activates our parasympathetic nervous system. This system controls our relaxation response and is what helps us to calm down in stressful situations. Breathing deeply is one of the best ways to lower stress in our bodies. It allows more oxygen to enter the bloodstream. It effectively quiets parts of the brain (including the amygdala), which then pass on messages to the body to relax by lowering heart rate and blood pressure.

You are probably, and understandably unconscious of the way you are breathing, but generally, there are two main types of breathing patterns:

- **Thoracic (chest) breathing**

Chest breathing happens during intense workouts or when one is in an emergency or scared. Most people subconsciously breathe this way naturally. When you lay on your back, place one hand on your chest and one hand on your stomach and breathe naturally. If your chest rises with each inhale, then you are a chest breather. This type of breathing can increase anxiety and make your muscles overly tense. When we become anxious, we tend to breathe rapidly with very shallow breaths at the top of our chest. Thoracic breathing stops your blood from being oxygenated properly and sends signals to your brain to activate the stress response. This is a large contributor to bringing on panic and anxiety attacks.

- **Diaphragmatic (abdominal) breathing**

[1]While lying down, place your hands as mentioned previously. If your belly pushes your hand outward while inhaling, then you are an abdominal breather. Breathing this way allows oxygen to move into the lungs and down through your abdomen, causing a relaxing response. When we are anxious, we must become aware of our breath to switch our breathing from thoracic to diaphragmatic consciously.

During a panic attack, you may experience symptoms such as headaches, visual changes, shaking or tingling, chest pain, and nausea. When we breathe too quickly, deeply, or irregularly, these symptoms are bound to happen, which sends a stress signal to the brain and causes the fight-or-flight response. The fight-or-flight response causes us to subconsciously breathe with our chests because our amygdala has sensed some form of threat and changes our breathing pattern so we can flee or prepare for combat.

With that said, there are techniques to help us notice when you are chest breathing, such as daily meditation and mindfulness, and switch to diaphragmatic breathing. When we experience panic attacks, we sometimes lose all control and forget everything we know about anxiety and coping methods, including breathing. This chapter will help bring your attention back to your breath and help you realize that you are only experiencing anxiety and nothing is wrong. So let's take a quick moment to practice diaphragmatic breathing.

STEP ONE:

1. Sit or lay down in a comfortable position.
2. Close your eyes and place your hands on your belly and your chest.
3. Ensure the surface you are sitting on has a backrest, as this exercise without daily practice can make you dizzy at first.

STEP TWO:

Breathe naturally (regardless of whether you are a chest or abdominal breather). Bring your attention to your breath. Notice where it is coming from. Become curious and mindful of where your breath comes from. Notice how fast or slow your breathing is. Notice how hot or cold your breath is. In this step, you are becoming present with yourself and your breath. Do not change the pace or force your breath. Let it happen naturally.

STEP THREE:

Relax your shoulders, and make sure your hands are in place. On your next inhale, push your belly hand outward as you breathe in, encouraging your stomach to rise with it. When you breathe out, your belly hand should sink in, and your chest hand should not move. If there is a slight movement with your chest hand, that is okay, notice this and repeat this process. Inhale and push your belly hand outward. Exhale and let your belly hand flatten while your chest hand remains still. Do this for as long as you need until you feel calmer and more relaxed.

AND YOU'RE DONE! WE HAVE JUST COMPLETED OUR FIRST breathing exercise. Abdominal breathing like that allows our bodies to become relaxed and comfortable so we can think rationally about our next move. It only takes a few moments, so we can do this at any time of the day. I recommend you do this every day, even when you don't experience panic attacks so that you can begin breathing this way subconsciously. Did you know that there are two types of ways to do breathing exercises? One way is 'in the moment' breathing, when we practice the exercise in the middle of whatever we're doing, the other is 'out of the moment' breathing. That is when we practice some form of daily meditation or guided breathing exercises when we are calm and not experiencing panic or anxiety.

IN THE MOMENT BREATHING TECHNIQUES

In the moment breathing is helpful to practice when we experience panic attacks and need to calm down immediately. Luckily there are many breathing techniques to choose from to know what works the best. Here are three 'in the moment' techniques you can try.

- **Box or Square Breathing**

[2]In chapter two, I briefly explained how box breathing works to calm your amygdala and help your prefrontal cortex take the lead. Square breathing heightens performance and helps you become focused. Athletes, Navy SEALS, police officers, therapists, and many doctors swear by this technique as it can instantly calm our nerves and give us the boost we need to carry on through our stressful days.

STEP ONE:

1. Choose a comfortable seating position where your feet are flat on the ground.
2. Let your hands fall naturally on your lap.

3. Sit straight, opening your belly, and aligning your neck with your spine.
4. Take in a couple of natural breaths and slowly switch your breath to diaphragmatic breathing.

Step Two:

When you are ready and are breathing with your belly, close your eyes. If it helps to become aware of your abdomen, place one hand on your belly and one on your chest, as previously mentioned. Let all your breath escape your lungs until you feel that you need to take an inhale immediately. On your next inhale, move to step three.

Step Three:

Inhale slowly through your nose, noticing your belly push outward, and count to four. As you do this, notice the air filling your lungs and belly. When you count to four, you are making sure that you are slowly counting. For example, one… missis…ippeee… Two… missis…ippee…

Step Four:

Hold your breath for the same slow count of four.

. . .

STEP FIVE:

Exhale through pursed lips (like blowing out a candle) for the same slow count of four. You are letting out all your breath in this step, making sure that your breath does not release quicker than your previous inhale. Become mindful of your anxiety symptoms disappearing. Feel the air leave your lungs.

STEP SIX:

Before taking in another breath, hold for a slow count of four. Once you have finished your count, repeat steps two through six ten more times or until you feel calmer.

While this may make you dizzy or lightheaded, *Mayo Clinic* suggests that if you breathe intentionally like this, it can lower your blood pressure and increase the amount of oxygen and carbon dioxide in your blood. The reason you feel calm and more relaxed after box breathing is because this buildup of CO_2 in your blood strengthens your vagus nerve when you exhale, which stimulates your parasympathetic system, resulting in your body becoming looser and less tense. While there are many benefits to box breathing and it's very helpful for calming an anxiety attack, beginners may experience uncomfortable symptoms. The more you practice, the easier it will become. However, if you become too dizzy or uncomfortable, return to your natural breath and try again from where you left off.

- **4-7-8 Breathing Exercise**

[3]With this exercise, it is best to have a place where you can lay down, as breathing this way is forceful and can be uncomfortable the first few times you do it. The 4-7-8 technique is like a natural tranquilizer to the nervous system. During an anxiety attack, the 4-7-8 breathing instantly alerts your fight-or-flight response team and tells it to go to sleep. This technique is excellent for helping us get to sleep and ridding us of the daily tension in our bodies that we have built up due to stress.

STEP ONE: RELEASE ALL YOUR BREATH ON YOUR EXHALE, making a whooshing sound with your mouth.

STEP TWO: CLOSE YOUR MOUTH AND BREATHE IN through your nose for a silent count of four. Make sure you are breathing in nice and slowly.

STEP THREE: ONCE YOU HAVE GOTTEN ALMOST A FULL breath through your nose, hold it for seven seconds. Try to count slowly. If you cannot hold your breath for seven the first couple of times you do this breathing exercise, go down to six, or wherever you feel comfortable.

STEP FOUR: SLOWLY EXHALE FOR A SILENT COUNT OF

eight through your mouth, as if you are blowing out birthday candles. Make sure your exhale is longer than both your inhale and hold points.

STEPS ONE THROUGH FOUR IS ONE BREATH. YOU WILL want to repeat this at least four times to feel the full effects of relaxation and decreased anxiety. This type of 'in the moment' breathing exercise can make you lightheaded the first few times you do it. Unlike the last breathing exercise, you should feel the effects of calmness almost instantly rather than having to practice at it every time you feel panicked.

- **Alternate Nasal Breathing**

Nasal breathing is a technique you learn when you practice yoga. It promotes clarity, instant anxiety relief, will power, and alertness. You can practice this technique right before a meeting or during an oncoming anxiety attack. Alternate nasal breathing requires you to plug one side of your nostril while breathing and then switching to the other side. When you breathe through your right nostril, you are connecting yourself to your personal nurturing energy. When you breathe through your left nostril, you are connecting yourself to cleansing energy.

STEP ONE:

1. Get into what's called the *Easy Pose* – cross your legs and keep your back and spine upright. Your left hand should rest on your left knee, connecting the index finger to your thumb.
2. Before you begin, close your eyes and focus on the middle of your forehead (third eye).
3. Relax.

STEP TWO: BRING YOUR RIGHT THUMB TO YOUR RIGHT nostril and inhale through your left nostril. Your mouth should be closed, and your belly should be pushing outward as you breathe in.

STEP THREE: LET GO OF YOUR RIGHT NOSTRIL, PLUG YOUR left with your index finger and exhale slowly. Let all the air escape your lungs and abdomen. Then, while still holding your left nostril, take a breath in once you have fully exhaled. Take a full, deep breath.

STEP FOUR: NOW, ALTERNATE YOUR INDEX FINGER TO your thumb, closing the right nostril on your exhale. It would be best if you exhale all your breath through the left nostril now. Before taking another deep breath in, switch your thumb back to your index, plugging the left and inhaling through your right nostril. Repeat these steps another fifteen times or until you feel calmer and more at ease.

Alternate nasal breathing like this helps lower your blood pressure and activates your parasympathetic nerve system, which tells your brain and amygdala that you are safe, and there is no threat. You can do this exercise before bed or when you're experiencing fluttering-like feelings brought on by anxiety.

There are many types of 'in the moment' breathing techniques that you can find online or on Youtube. However, the previous exercises are for when you need immediate relief or cannot get to sleep. Let's now take a look at what you can do actively every day when you do not experience panic and anxiety.

OUT OF THE MOMENT BREATHING TECHNIQUES

Out of the moment breathing is when you practice some form of daily meditation or guided breathing exercises when you are calm and not experiencing panic or anxiety. These meditations can be practiced at any time of day, but many people like to practice at night when they are ready to fall asleep. A good example of this is mindfulness meditation.

MINDFULNESS MEDITATION

[4]Mindfulness is practiced to gain self-awareness and emotional resiliency. In a mindfulness meditation, we focus only on the breath and we are encouraged to notice our thoughts and bodily sensations without judging or labeling them. Remember thinking traps? Mindfulness allows us to see these thoughts for what they are rather than blowing them up and reacting to them.

In this mindfulness exercise, you will not force your breaths or count them; you are merely noticing your breath and sensations.

STEP ONE:

1. Relax in a seated or lying down position.
2. Make sure you are comfortable and in a quiet setting where you will not be disturbed.
3. Close your eyes, and take a few breaths.

STEP TWO:

While inhaling, notice where your breath is coming from. Is it your chest, belly, nose, or multiple places? Is your breath cold or hot? As you exhale, notice how fast or slow your breath is. Notice your heartbeat. Is it thumping hard in your chest, or can you barely feel it?

STEP THREE:

1. Keep focusing on your breath. If your mind happens to wander elsewhere, notice this and bring your attention back to your breath.
2. Become curious as you breathe in and out naturally.
3. Continue to breathe and start to bring your attention to other parts of your body.

What does the surface below you feel like? Soft, hard, cold, warm? What is your stomach doing? Notice any tingling or bodily sensations you may be experiencing. Without judgment, notice your feelings as neutral, then return to your breath.

STEP FOUR:

Notice your breath again. Has it changed pace, or does it remain the same as when you started? Now, bring your attention to your thoughts. Remember, your thoughts are just thoughts. Your feelings are just feelings. You are not labeling them as good, bad, happy, or sad. You are not judging them as anxious or traumatic. Notice whatever thought that pops in your head and then bring your attention to your breath again. Inhale. Exhale. Inhale and exhale.

Mindfulness helps you become aware of yourself, but mostly on your breath. Your thoughts will often wander, but that is why you bring your focus back to your breath; to become present with this particular moment.

MANTRA MEDITATION

This type of meditation uses a word, phrase, or sound to help relax the mind and body. As a beginner, the mantra you use may not have much of an effect; however, with practice, over time, you will become instantly relaxed when you hear or say this mantra. The mantra can be spoken aloud or quietly.

STEP ONE: AFTER FINDING A RESTFUL PLACE TO GET settled, close your eyes and take a deep breath in and a deep breath out (as if you are sighing). Steady your breath and become in tune with it.

STEP TWO: THINK OF A MANTRA. THIS COULD BE ONE word such as 'relax' or one phrase such as 'I am here.' Or, if you would prefer sound, think of a sound that calms you, like a bell dinging every three seconds or water dripping rhythmically from a tap. If you are more of a visual individual, you can picture a candle flame flickering slightly or a blade of grass blowing in the wind.

STEP THREE: WITH EVERY INHALE, REPEAT YOUR MANTRA once and then exhale. Inhale, say, listen to, or visualize your mantra, and exhale slowly. For example, breathe in slowly, say, 'I am safe,' and now breathe out. Inhale and say, 'I am safe,' and exhale.

AND THAT'S IT. MANTRA MEDITATION NOT ONLY HELPS US relax; it helps us become more aware of ourselves when we are anxious or heightened. Over time, during a panicky situation, you can repeat this mantra, and you will feel that all your anxious symptoms seem to disappear almost instantly.

PROGRESSIVE RELAXATION

This type of meditation is also known as the body scan. It requires you to breathe in deeply and start from your head and work down to your toes. You are tightening the small group of muscles in each area as you breathe in, and as you exhale, you are releasing the tension. The body scan helps you understand what individual body parts feel like when they tense up as opposed to what they feel like when we are relaxed. It will help you understand how constricted you feel during an anxiety attack, so you don't have to guess whether it's anxiety, or something is actually wrong. Once you know this feeling by heart, you will know when you can do 'in the moment' breathing exercises. We will only go through the first few steps, as progressive relaxation is a long process.

STEP ONE:

1. Ensure you are lying flat on your back, legs, and arms not touching your body.
2. Close your eyes, and focus your attention on your face.
3. Breathe in slowly and deeply while also scrunching your face together.
4. Imagine you are trying to push your entire face onto your nose.
5. Exhale, and return your face to normal and relaxed.

STEP TWO:

On your next deep inhale, notice your shoulders and scrunch them up to your ears, flex your arms and hold while you breathe in. This may not be easy, but as you practice, it will get easier. Exhale and release all tension. Relax fully on your exhale.

.   .   .

STEP THREE:

Continue working through each body part as you inhale and exhale through the exercise. Next will be your hands and fingers, then your chest, stomach, back, buttocks, thighs, calves, ankles, and toes. As you work through each body part, notice the difference between constricted and relaxed.

During this exercise, some people choose to go from their toes to their heads, while others choose one side then work up the other side of their body. You can play around with this exercise and choose what is most comfortable for you. This type of meditation aims to unwind and de-stress us entirely before falling asleep or doing a stressful activity.

[5]There are many different meditation exercises to choose from, each bringing their own benefits and goals. Meditation not only creates resilience to stress and anxiety but continues to instill long-term benefits for our entire lives. It's like the gift that keeps on giving that only you can give to yourself. Mostly, the goal is to shift our attention from the busyness of our own lives to a non-judgmental tranquil perception. Eventually, after practicing with meditation, we will become more focused, self-aware, and emotionally tolerant. These skills are great to cultivate in our lives because we feel better physically, emotionally, and spiritually.

CHAPTER SUMMARY

While breathing is a subconscious act we don't usually worry about in our daily lives, teaching ourselves to breathe with our diaphragm rather than with our chest will ultimately calm our anxious nerves. Practicing these exercises in the moment and out of the moment will permanently dial down our amygdalas' fight-or-flight response, resulting in fewer panic attacks and decreased anxiety when we feel stressed. Most of these exercises take time, practice, and dedication to see results, but if you stick with the habit, you will see significant results.

As a reminder, in this chapter, we learned;

- Panic attack breathing techniques
- Meditation exercises to practice daily
- Why breathing with our diaphragm brings on less anxiety
- Why chest breathers feel more anxious

In the next chapter, you will learn how to bring everything you learned thus far into your daily lives and make each coping mechanism a habit so that you can start to feel positive differences.

7

COMMIT TO LONG-TERM HABITS

Now it's time to make these new habits stick for the long term. This chapter will help you to identify;

- What behavior spotters are and how they are beneficial
- What your barriers are and how to fix them.
- What to do if you fall off track
- How to accomplish the small things to boost dopamine and serotonin
- How to make sleep and exercise a part of your everyday habit
- How to change sleeping habits

How many times do we try to establish long-term habits, whether they be to exercise daily, eat healthier, sleep better, meditate daily, etc.? Unfortunately, as we've all found, habits are incredibly hard to form. However, to ensure healthy mental health, we can create new habits to better our lives and become successful in our future goals – aka, less or no anxiety. It is no understatement to say your mental health has to be a priority in your life. The habits to achieve this need to be simple, achievable, and measurable in some way. In this chapter, I want to talk about habits that I found incredibly helpful for my mental health and simple to implement.

ENLIST BEHAVIOR SPOTTERS

This is difficult to start with, but it asks us to tell people when we are anxious. By talking to people around us when we feel anxious, they can help us identify patterns and behaviors that we adopt when we're becoming anxious, which can help identify when our anxiety brains are taking the lead. The sooner we can recognize the changes in our behavior, the earlier we will identify when to interrupt the anxious brain thought processes and almost stop them before they begin. I have a close circle of people around me who notice when my behavior changes and I become a 'less vibrant' version of myself. Sometimes they get it wrong, and I am just feeling overwhelmed! But more often than not, they are right, and I can catch it early before I get into an anxious spiral.

Some of the patterns my *spotters* monitor are:

1. Nausea and reduced appetite
2. Overanalyzing conversations to confirm a negative outcome
3. Struggling to fall asleep or waking early
4. Inability to sustain concentration

You might identify different patterns, but by noting them, writing them down, and sharing them with people close to you, you will be able to spot them early and implement the hacks in chapter three quickly.

IDENTIFYING BARRIERS

Forming new habits can be uncomfortable to start because they take planning, recognizing when we have slipped up, and persistently driving to keep them going. The goal for habits is to get them to become as comfortable and automatic as breathing. It can be tough to make changes when we are already so used to doing what we have always done. So, it takes resilience, self-awareness, and motivation to make and continue with the change you need. Before we dive into creating a schedule to develop some new habits, let's take a look at what barriers we might come up against first.

Barrier number one: 'I forgot.'

It's easy to forget a new habit when we are just starting

because it's something new we have to become aware of. A few things we can try for the sake of remembering are:

- Write our habits in a daily planner
- Post sticky notes where our habit takes place
- Download a habit tracker app

After seeing your sticky notes every day or hearing a notification coming from your phone every day, you will get used to following your habit. Eventually, you won't need the reminders.

Barrier number two: 'I am overwhelmed with all this change. I have too many habits on the go.'

For most people, we get an idea in our heads and then become so excited that we start doing everything all at once. It's like starting new projects such as learning to crochet or taking up painting. We find ourselves putting all our time and energy into these things for about a week, then we slowly stop and get back into our old routine. So, when it comes to building new habits for our mental health, starting slowly and keeping it interesting will help us push forward and keep it at a steady pace. Some things that can keep us on track without feeling overwhelmed are:

- Starting one habit a week (or every two weeks, your own pace).
- Focus on habits that work together, such as journaling and then meditating right after. Or:

○ Exercising then showering
○ Brushing your teeth, then flossing
○ Meditating then sleeping

- Try switching one habit for the new one, such as:

  ○ Switching coffee for tea
  ○ Watching TV for journaling
  ○ Playing phone games for reading
  ○ Laying down for sitting straight and moving
     your legs on an exercise ball
  ○ Driving down the road for walking or biking
     down the road

When we switch old habits for new ones, it makes it easier for our brains to understand that we are doing something different. With practice, we will automatically start developing new habits without noticing much, then those old habits will become history, and we can move onto more meaningful goals. If we combine our new habits with another new habit, we teach our brains what we feel comfortable doing together, therefore resulting in a new comfort zone.

Barrier number three: 'I gave up.' Or 'I gave in to my temptation.'

Let's say that these new habits are starting to work, but then we become lazy one day, and nothing terrible happens. So, we think, *'Well, if nothing bad happened and I skipped my habit for the day, then it's not so bad, and I don't need to contin-*

ue." Next thing we know, a week goes by, and we are back to experiencing anxiety and feelings of panic out of nowhere. Now we're thinking, *'Oh no, where did I go wrong?'* This is called giving in to temptation, whether wanting to skip the habit or deciding that we're fine without it. So, how can we conquer these temptations?

- Figure out the temptation behind the habit.
  Examples:

  - Exercise – Feeling lazy or not into it
  - Changing diet – The old diet is tastier
  - Journaling – Don't feel like it, hands hurt
  - Meditating – It's too dull
  - Sleep – Rather be awake and think

- Change the time of day or setting.

  - Exercise – Switch from morning to night or vice versa. Go outside or stay at home
  - Meditation – Figure out the best time of day to do this that fits with your schedule
  - Journaling – What time of day and where in your house are you most inspired?
  - Sleep – Have you finished all that you need to do before you're ready for some shut-eye? Try journaling

- Make the habit more inviting than the temptation. Example:

  - Exercise – Try sleeping in your workout clothes, so it's one less thing you have to do in the morning
  - Meditation – Decorate your meditation area with tranquil sounds and inviting scents
  - Journaling – Create a place for a mini-office. Reward yourself with books, writing utensils, or buy computer software if you prefer to type
  - Sleep – Sleep on the couch. Set up a tent in your backyard with a mini fire and go backyard camping

The idea is to figure out the problem, ask yourself questions about your temptations, and then solve it by creating greater rewards for your new habit than the temptation you're resisting.

While many barriers come our way when we start new habits to better ourselves, every barrier may sound somewhat similar to the three I mentioned above. The goal is to find the problem and change the way we are making the habit, or the place we are trying to create our habit in. This is why it's beneficial to have a buddy who wants to create similar life changes like you. Together, you can identify each other's barriers and help each other push past them.

WHAT HAPPENS IF I FALL OFF TRACK?

[1]So you started working on the habit(s) for a little while, but then somewhere along the way, you fell off track, and you're just noticing now what feels like months later. You might be thinking, '*Where did I go wrong?*' Before we succumb to our thinking traps and become super negative, stop – Pat yourself on the back for even realizing that you have fallen off track. Look at the positive. Just because we have strayed from a routine we were trying to implement doesn't mean we need to give up altogether. When this happens, take a look at your barriers, review how habits are formed (explained back in chapter four), and restart your habit-forming plan.

See this as an opportunity to journal, to write down what you are feeling at this point. Write down what you were trying to do before you slipped, when you noticed and when you remember the last time you practiced your new habits, and then create a plan to move forward. If you have notes from what you were doing previously, take a moment to read these over to get back on track. The thing about creating new habits is that sometimes they don't fall into place with our lifestyles. So, we have two options.

- A – Change our lifestyle to fit our habits
- B – Change our habits to suit our lifestyle

Option B is usually the easier way to do things since our lives are always changing, and new things are always happening around us. Whether we are attending our best friend's wedding, which takes up our time or finding out we are pregnant or someone we know is. Anything can happen instantly, which is why it can be challenging to change our lifestyle or implement new habits in our lives. Also, we all have those days where we just aren't feeling into doing anything. While this is okay, it's best not to create a habit of procrastinating and continue putting things off. So let's start from the beginning:

- **Identify why you started this new habit**

The reason behind the habit is your winning ticket. It's the motivation behind your success. If we're making a habit just because someone else told us to try, then we're most likely bound to fail. However, if we are doing it because we want to see change, opportunity, and to work on ourselves, that is enough reason to continue pushing forward. By the way, journal the reasons for your new habit in your habit tracker or planner so that you can return to these reasons for motivation on those 'off' days. The reason has to be good enough for you so that you can return to the habit and say, 'I want this'.

- **Create a schedule for your habit(s)**

Jotting your habit down into your calendar or daily planner means that that spot in your schedule is reserved, so now you have to plan around it. This is one way you can use option A to implement your habit into your life, by changing your lifestyle to support your growing habit. Now that this has been penciled in, try doing this at the same time every day. Over time, you will start to recognize what you are doing before you start your new habit and what you feel afterward, ultimately resulting in a successful routine.

- **Go over your barriers again**.

Take a look at the barriers I mentioned. Can you think of any other barriers that lead you to fall off track? Write these down, and figure out a solution. Eventually, you will fight against all your barriers, and your habit will become automatically structured inside your mind so that you don't fall off the wagon again.

- **Call up your behavior spotters and habit buddies**.

Remember the behavior spotters I mentioned previously? I strongly recommend you find one of your own if you haven't already. These habit buddies are here to support and help us when we fall. Make sure it's someone you like to hang out with, someone you can connect with, and someone who knows what you are trying to do. We want all the support we can get.

- **Start small**

Failing is part of success because it helps us learn where we went wrong. So in actuality, did you fail, or did you learn to become more resilient? Going back to the beginning of how we form habits, they all start with a cue, then a craving, the response to the craving or trigger, and finally a reward. So if we're trying to start our habit of meditating, we would start small by first figuring out what time of day we want to feel relaxed or more focused. This could be before work or before we lay down to fall asleep. The cue would be feeling tense; the craving would be to want to feel calmer; the response would be to meditate actively. The reward is feeling relaxed and more secure. Now do this every day at the same time, and you have just mastered your first daily habit.

- **Create a new environment**

With change comes difficult choices. If you want to implement a workout habit, but none of your friends are active and don't want to exercise, then it's time to make some new friends to work out with. However, this is an easy one because you can go down to the gym and start working out around other active people. Conversations will start, and new relationships will form.

If you want to start a habit of getting a better night's sleep, it is worth considering your surroundings. Scan your bedroom and figure out what is contributing to the lack of sleep structure you're getting. It could be that it's too hot, too stuffy, your bed is too hard or soft, your partner snores too loud, or you have a TV in your room. It could be anything. When starting a new habit, take a look at your environment and change it accordingly.

It's always more comfortable to do things we are used to, so starting new habits takes time and effort to master and enjoy. But that's just it. The habits we are trying to implement into our lives must be things we enjoy doing. And if they aren't, we must start small with no pressure to do the entire routine. For example, when starting an exercise routine, you cannot expect to wake up and enjoy a one-mile run. First, you start with climbing the stairs a couple of times, followed by stretching. Start at the bottom and what is most comfortable, then climb to the top. Keep a journal entry of almost everything you do so that you can identify patterns of what works and what doesn't.

Most importantly, be compassionate and understanding with yourself. Often, we put too much pressure on ourselves to do what we expect of ourselves without really looking at what is realistic. So if you fall, get back up and try again. No harm was done. If you don't feel like it, do something small and simple. Just because you didn't follow through with the entire habit doesn't mean you didn't at least try to start it.

HOW DO I BOOST MY DOPAMINE AND SEROTONIN WITH ALL THIS HABIT AND CHANGE?

I always have a goal on the go. My goal right now is to write this book, but previous ones have been; complete an online course, run three times a week for three months, and listen to a new podcast every week. I find it useful to have a section in my journal where I jot down goal ideas as they come to me. Then I can filter through them and create an action plan for them when I start. The online course is a good one as they do all the preparation and planning for you...and you get something at the end!

Practically, as I go through my list, I write down the steps to accomplish my goal. With every step that I complete, I reward myself, which boosts my dopamine hormones, and I feel good about myself. As I said, my current goal is writing this book right now, but it would be overwhelming to write the entire thing in one sitting. Now, every day that I have accomplished even one paragraph, I congratulate myself, and that makes me feel good.

[2]Setting milestones every step of the way and achieving them little by little not only helps boost serotonin but helps us see how far we have come from when we started. Everything I mentioned in this chapter thus far boosts our feel-good hormones, resulting in dialing down our stress hormones and living a less anxiety-filled life. So, let's look into how we can

change our sleeping routine and create a healthy exercise plan that works.

HOW TO MAKE EXERCISE A PART OF YOUR DAILY ROUTINE

[3]Since we discussed how exercise is crucial to combatting and fighting off our stress hormones, resulting in decreased anxiety and increased resilience to stressful situations, I thought exercise must be our top priority to tackle. Alongside sleep, of course.

- **Become curious for the first week**

When starting your first habit of a workout routine, it's best to write down what you think you will enjoy. Some activities include:

- Walking in nature
- Working on strength and toning at the gym
- Yoga
- Bike riding
- Jogging

For the first week, do something different every day. By the end of the week, you will know what you enjoy and what you don't. Next week, plan your routine starting out small and deciding a daily milestone to a more significant weekly milestone and follow it for three months. Remember to reward yourself after each goal has been completed.

- **Establish a workout buddy and a behavior spotter**

I cannot stress this enough! Have a support team behind you. The benefit of having someone alongside you is that they can watch for when your behavior or mood starts to change and work at helping you change it. You will also feel more energized and motivated if you're not feeling 'alone' through this new change. Besides, having someone to socialize with and support back boosts your dopamine levels because not only are you getting the support and encouragement you need, you are also responsible for helping them.

- **Figure out which environment and what time of day works best for you**

It can be challenging to find the right time that works for you. I am a morning person, so working out or exercising at this time helps me stay focused and motivated to want to exercise. You could be the same, or you could be the opposite, so it's best to find this out and then implement your new routine in your life. If you are a morning person, try to wake up earlier than expected and hit the gym before heading to work. Not only will this set you up for success throughout your day due to your increased dopamine and concentration, but you will also feel a new sense of accomplishment. If you're more of a night owl, then getting a nightly stroll in your neighborhood will help you become restful and relaxed, setting you up for a good night's sleep.

- **Exercise during a barrier episode**

Since exercise is a great natural feel-good hormone inducer, exercising through your barriers will increase dopamine and serotonin, making you feel a lot better than you did. You will feel the difference in your mood, energy, and overall resilience to stressful events. What you thought was a big deal will seem like molehills the more you exercise through your barriers.

- **After each workout, jot it down in a workout journal**

Keeping a workout journal helps you stay focused and curious. Jot down what you did, how you felt before, during, and after, then what your goal is for next time. This will also help you keep track of your milestones and become closer to your big reward. After a couple of weeks or a month goes by, you can reread through your workout journal and see the differences you have felt since you started. You may have felt tired and unmotivated when you started, but as you go on, you are noticing you're getting a full night's rest, your mood is better, you're having more clarity, and most importantly, you have less anxiety during the day.

Part of starting a new workout routine means that you must never forget about rewarding yourself. Each habit begins with a cue and ends with a reward. So after about a week of exercising, you may feel sore from using muscles you never even knew you had, but the reward after your milestone makes it all worth it, not to mention how you will feel, how you will think, and what you will experience during your journey. Don't worry if you slip up or fall off track. The fact that you have failed means that you didn't fail; you just learned something new and can notice it quicker next time.

HOW TO CHANGE YOUR SLEEP HABITS TO GET A BETTER NIGHT'S REST

[4]Insomnia is a frustrating cycle. First, we feel exhausted, but as soon as we lay down, it's like we could run an entire marathon right now. Our minds are distracting us with everything we must do tomorrow or everything we haven't done today. Our bodies are fidgety because we're not ready to relax yet. If it's not one thing we try and fail at, it's another. The problem is we overthink when it's time to sleep. We put so much pressure on ourselves to will ourselves sleep that it just doesn't happen. Before we know it, the sun is peeping through our windows, and we might as well get up because it's not going to happen. Now we find ourselves forcing productivity throughout the day, or we become daily daydreamers.

So, let's look at a few things we can do to stop this pattern from even happening:

- **Change your sleep environment.**

Take a look at your bedroom. Ensure that it feels homey and safe as this is one thing we connect our energy to – the vibe a room gives off. If you have painful memories in your bedroom, put some positive pictures on the wall, and redecorate. Arrange your room so that your bed is somewhere new, you don't have a TV calling out your name at night, and your phone is across the room from your bed; so that you have to get up to look at it but don't because you are warm and comfy. Place your bed under or by a window, so you get a draft, making it easier to breathe through the night. Maybe invest in an anxiety blanket (that can be a reward for creating a bedtime routine and sticking with it). Make the room that you sleep in as comforting and relaxing as you can. Instead of getting rid of all electronics right off the bat, try replacing your TV with a music device so that you can listen to relaxing sounds while you try to sleep.

- **Write in your journal**

Our journals are there for us to jot all our thoughts, emotions, and stressors in. So, have one placed by your bed or under your pillow with a pen if you wake through the night and need to jot something else down like your dream. Get everything out so that there is nothing left to think about. Even if one word pops into your mind, write this down too. Then, when you're trying to sleep, if anything else pops in your mind, you have the journal close by that you can quickly jot that in. This tells your brain that you aren't ignoring the thoughts, but you are writing them down and dealing with them later. You are essentially creating a 'worry box' where you write everything down and then come back to it later if it still bothers you at a better time.

- **Choose a Meditation**

I suggest any one of the previous 'out of the moment' exercises mentioned in the last chapter. My favorite is mindfulness meditation. It helps settle my mind, my body, and all my nerves so that I can sink into my blankets with no worries and no stress. Sometimes, if I am lucky, I will fall asleep before my meditation is finished. It helps when you listen to guided meditations so that you aren't distracted by your voice and personal memories brought up during the exercise. Although you may have memories or thoughts distracting you from the guided exercise, you can at least notice them quicker and return your focus to the person speaking to you.

- **Create a 'same time every day' nightly routine**

Set the alarm about an hour before you want to go to sleep. This will give you enough time to finish what you're doing and follow through with your nightly schedule. Make sure whatever your nightly schedule is, you do this at the same time every single night. It is essential to keep this up at least in the beginning because you are rewiring and training your brain to do and follow through with something new and different. Over time, you can switch it up and do what feels more natural to you, but we want to create a base structure for you to follow.

- **Still can't sleep? Change scenery.**

Even after all that, you still cannot sleep? Get up and get a light snack, go outside and breathe some fresh air, and try again. Sometimes, all it takes is a little change in scenery and an excuse for your mind to become slightly distracted before it's ready to prepare for sleep.

During your new sleep habit, make sure that you avoid caffeinated beverages and switch to nighttime teas such as chamomile, peppermint, or valerian root. Avoid eating heavy meals, rather stick to light snacks like yogurt, a slice of bread, or cheese and crackers. If you have opted for sleep aids such as vitamins or supplements earlier discussed, and you have talked to your doctor, feel free to take these about half an hour before you intend to lay down. Sleep triggers the natural melatonin in our brains and vice versa. It is up to us to induce the melatonin hormone by engaging in relaxing activities and ensuring that our sleep surroundings are comfortable and secure.

CHAPTER SUMMARY

Creating new habits is one of the biggest challenges you will face on this journey to overcoming anxiety. However, the in this chapter we looked at how you can be successful and stay on track! Remember to;

- Set habitual milestones and reward your achievements to increase the feel-good factor
- Take exercise and commit to a sleep schedule to build resilience to stress
- Set up a buddy system and get behavior spotter onboard
- Fight off those habit barriers

8

PULLING IT ALL TOGETHER

In this chapter we will review and solidify:

- What normal anxiety is vs disordered anxiety
- How we can combat bad feelings and put ourselves first
- How to boost our 'feel good' chemicals in everyday routines

For some people, anxiety is so intense that it disrupts our daily lives, which makes it hard to stay positive and feel almost 'normal'. We get so lost in our anxiety/thinking traps that we see everything as either negative, black and white, or super dangerous as if something terrible is going to happen. Over time, the more we think and believe the irrational thoughts our amygdala is telling us, we start to block out our rational

mind – the prefrontal cortex – which results in physical feelings of being on edge and continuously revved up.

Throughout this book, you have learned strategies for challenging your anxious brain and how to create new habits to
build resilience to anxiety. We often look at anxiety as a bad
thing because of the symptoms we experience during an
attack. However, anxiety is not something to be ashamed of,
nor is it something we should be scared of. Anxiety is very
normal human response behavior. Anxiety can also be beneficial during an intensely traumatic event such as a car accident
or a less traumatic but still alarming event such as when we
take a shortcut home at night, walking through a dark alley.
This is when our instincts and overactive mind should be on
alert. Still, once we escape the potentially dangerous situation,
our anxiety should fade, and we go on as typically as we
normally would. However, for anxiety sufferers like us, we
experience panic and adrenaline even after we have come from
walking in a dark alley or weeks after a traumatic event.

Anxiety disorder is a recognized medical condition, and it
is important that we take care of ourselves just as we would
with any illness. Sometimes that means putting our needs
before others'.

PUTTING YOURSELF FIRST

[1]The first way to climb out of the anxiety hole is to treat yourself with compassion and put yourself and your health above
all else. While this may sound selfish or self-centered, you

mustn't believe that myth. Selfishness is when you are engaged with others to get what you need and don't think about what they need or what you could give back. Putting yourself first means that you are making an effort to take care of yourself and replenish your own needs because you know that you are just as important as other people. You are ensuring your needs are met without taking away from others.

Before we recap about the strategies we can use to put ourselves first, let's look at why you may feel like you can't.

- **We think people will judge us**

When we are so used to putting others before ourselves, we get stuck in this trap of always helping someone and regularly forgetting about ourselves. Then we begin to think if we start cherishing ourselves or buying ourselves gifts and rewarding ourselves, then the people we used to do that for will stop liking us.

The truth is that people who love us will understand when we want to make a difference in our own lives as much as theirs. If they don't, then maybe it's time to look at your inner circle and reconsider who is worth your time rather than whether you are worth the time of others.

- **We would rather sacrifice to make someone else happy**

Helping others boosts our dopamine and serotonin, which

ultimately makes us feel good, because when we help others and take care of other people, the feel-good receptors in our brains light up.

The issue with this, though, is that even though we become happy, we can unintentionally become overwhelmed if we continually offer our caring services to others without reciprocation because we are slowly emptying our jug. So, essentially, what can you give if you run out of things to give? The only way you can look after others is if you are pleased about yourself. Your happy meter is full because you have spent time putting yourself first, too. Find a balance.

- **What if we miss out on something?**

Perhaps you feel as though if you put yourself first and work on lifting yourself, you will miss out on what everyone else is doing. Maybe you won't get invited to outings anymore, or maybe people won't want to hang out with you because they think you are too selfish.

The fact is that most people who share on their social media pages or discuss things about their lives publicly may have other things going on behind the scenes that we are entirely unaware of. Don't worry; you won't miss out on anything as long as you continue to enjoy your own life. The one thing that matters the most is not missing out on your own life while you're being distracted by everyone else's. If you feel like you're missing out, call up your friends that post on social media and check in. You never know how close you can get to someone if you make the first effort to become engaged. Also, a bonus fact is that the more sociability we have in our lives, the more our serotonin increases, resulting in less anxiety and a much happier day.

- **We feel that we may not deserve it**

The thing about anxiety is that it gets us to think cynically and then believe our own lies. You may think, 'I don't deserve to feel pretty.' Or 'I'm not worth my own time.' This way of thinking only creates a fire that feeds our anxious brains to keep us in a dull state. The more we continue to put others first, the more substantial the habit becomes to the point where putting ourselves first feels almost alien.

The fact is though, regardless of what our negative thoughts are trying to tell us, our obsessive nature to help and control things around us isn't helping ourselves. So, spending time with others that are positive, upbeat, and confident will show you that if they can do it, you are strong enough to put in the effort to feel happy too.

Whatever you tell yourself, there is always a more upbeat and positive solution, one being journaling and positive, uplifting affirmations. So, how do we get into the habit of putting ourselves first?

- Write personal notes and stick them everywhere in your house. Pick up some sticky notes from the dollar store or make some flashcards you can put

in your purse or wallet when you're out and about.
Make sure these sticky notes and flashcards have
affirmations such as:

- I am worth my time
- I have the strength to get through anything.
- I have been through worse, so this next task
  is nothing in comparison
- I am good enough
- I am healthy and resilient

- Journal gratitude. Writing down what you have
  and what you're thankful for can boost your mood
  when you're feeling anxious or depressed. Later,
  you can look at these statements and reassure
  yourself that you are rich by merely being grateful
  for all you have and all you worked towards.
  Bonus, creating an accomplishment journal helps
  increase your dopamine levels because you can
  then cross off and remember that you are actively
  creating a better life for yourself. Essentially this is
  putting yourself first.
- When you feel like you have failed, encourage
  yourself. Failure is only a state of mind if we sit
  there and stew on the fact that we did something
  wrong or haven't completed something we wanted
  to do. When you feel like you failed, look back at
  your sticky notes or flashcards and re-read what

you feel about yourself to lift you up. Then create an encouragement list. This list could include:

○ I didn't fail. I learned.
○ I didn't give up. I took a step back to push forward.
○ I didn't ignore my friend. I took a minute for myself – and that's allowed.
○ I didn't lose control. I faced my fear and pushed through.

• Become mindful in every stressful situation. Remember chapter six? Re-read the mindful exercise, and just take a quick moment for yourself to stay mindful at the moment. You can stay mindful during a bath, during a stressful activity, in the middle of a panic attack, or right before bed. Remember, all you are doing is noticing your breath and your body without labeling or becoming judgmental.

Doing these activities daily and making a conscious effort to implement them into your daily routine creates a dopamine and serotonin booster, which will help you become resilient towards anxiety and stress. One thing you may definitely want to try is to continue to forgive yourself if you think you have done something wrong. Holding onto grudges or overestimating your ability to cope can damage your mental health and increase the stress response more often. Let go of the baggage and create a growth type of mindset. When there is a problem, instead of thinking, 'Oh no, I have failed. I will never be xxx. I will always stay xxx,' say things like, 'Okay, so I ran into a speed bump, what can I do right now to solve this and make myself feel better?' If there is no solution, take a step back, write it out, or go over your affirmation cards. That way, you can subdue what your amygdala is trying to tell you and come back to it with your PFC later and come up with a resolution.

PERMANENTLY BOOST YOUR FEEL-GOOD HORMONES

[2]Remember chapter three and seven? These chapters explain the importance of serotonin and dopamine. Adequate amounts of sleep, regular exercise, relaxing activities, and positive self-talk contribute to boosting serotonin. Also, when we talked about habits; checking off our accomplishments once we achieved our daily milestones significantly increases our dopamine because it gives us a boost of confidence and self-esteem. Plus, it always feels good to reward ourselves with gifts or something we look forward to.

Here are some things you can do to boost your serotonin and dopamine hormones daily:

- **Diet**

Remember tryptophan? Tryptophan is found in foods that have high protein levels. Couple tryptophan with twenty-five to thirty grams of carbohydrates and watch your mood skyrocket from anxious to energized. Tryptophan helps induce the serotonin hormones so that you feel more relaxed and obtain more energy throughout the day. Also, try foods such as:

- A turkey sandwich on whole-wheat bread
- Peanut butter and crackers with a glass of milk
- Salmon or tuna with brown rice
- Oatmeal and nuts

- **Exercise**

Speaking of tryptophan, did you know that exercising daily can trigger the release of tryptophan entering your bloodstream? As a result, exercising allows the stability for tryptophan to enter your brain, ultimately making you feel good. These exercises can include:

- Swimming
- Yoga

- Brisk walking
- Jogging
- Hiking in nature

- **Vitamin D**

Go outside and breathe in the fresh air. It doesn't necessarily have to be sunny, but as long as you're being introduced
to bright light or natural light daily, your serotonin levels will
increase. Have you ever noticed how the weather has an effect
on your mood? Some people become more depressed in the
wintertime due to the lack of sunshine they get. So in the
winter months, make sure you pick up a Vitamin D bottle and
take this daily.

- **Vitamin B12**

Vitamin B12 is like a serotonin booster because it targets
our mood. Coupled with 5-HTP and tryptophan, it's like
getting a dose of sunshine without the sun! Vitamin B12 is
essential for our overall health, so before that jog, make sure to
take a vitamin B12 supplement or promise to eat some healthy
greens.

- **Massage**

Throughout the entire book, I have expressed the importance of rewarding yourself. One excellent way to reward your-

self for a significant milestone is to book yourself for a weekly or monthly massage. It helps increase serotonin, decreases cortisol levels, and helps you become more resilient to stress and anxiety. Something about massages makes us feel good anyways, but the feeling you get afterward when your muscles have completely relaxed and the only thing you're focused on is that feeling of your muscles and joints becoming loose. Ahhhhh, there is no better feeling than a massage.

- **Reminiscing happy memories**

So, maybe you are having a dark day, and it's just one of those days where you may be feeling extra anxious or super depressed for no apparent reason. Looking through a photo album or calling a friend will distract your mind from your day, and it will increase your serotonin levels almost immediately. Although it might not work as you intend it to right away, sometimes just bringing yourself to a happier situation like listening to happy music or engaging in a hobby you love can relax you enough to get out of that state of mind.

IF, FOR WHATEVER REASON, YOU FEEL AS THOUGH YOU can't get out of an anxious or depressed state, make sure you check in with your doctor periodically. He or she may refer you to a therapist who will help you identify any triggers you may not have known about. Seeking help through professionals can also increase dopamine and serotonin. The good thing about increasing your feel-good hormones is that it's easy to do as long as whatever you spend your time doing is positive, uplifting, and enjoyable for you. The higher these hormones are, the less your stress hormones come to disturb your life.

CHAPTER SUMMARY

So, where do we go from here?

It's important to remember that when you put yourself first, and engage in social and personal growth-type activities, your anxiety **will** reduce. When you actively do the things that make you feel good every day, your brain **will** anticipate positivity and **will** increase those anxiety busting hormones.

You have the knowledge and tools, you just have to go ahead and do it!

APPENDIX

If you jumped ahead to this chapter then let's get started with this super fast and effective action plan. It is only seven days long but it needs you to commit totally to it. Make sure all the important people in your life know you are doing it and you will need their support for the next seven days. You will be amazed by how much they want to help you! They will feel relieved they can be useful in helping you feel better.

Firstly, YOU have to take priority for the next week. Your job, family, friends, house all need to be secondary. It is the analogy of putting your own gas mask on first before you can help anyone else. If you don't prioritize yourself now, everything else will suffer. The goal behind this seven-day plan is to get used to change and build yourself a new habit so that you can become less anxious. This is why it must take your full attention and commitment.

You are the priority! Your health and wellbeing is the priority. You will be reading this thinking 'I can't be that self-ish' and 'Everyone is depending on me!' But this is the most selfless thing you will ever do. No one can depend or rely on you until you are well physically and mentally. Just think, if you had a broken leg, people would rally around and support you for at least six weeks! You are only engaged in this for one full week!.

Seriously, no excuses, your kids will be absolutely fine eating beans on toast and watching TV for one week. Think of this as your own personal vacation that you have longed for and deserved. Your boss can manage without you for seven days, just make sure you plan this ahead of time so that he or she is well aware and will grant you the time to work on yourself. Your house can gather dust for one week! It really isn't a big deal. The bigger issue will be if you don't take this time to get well.

If people around you see you investing in your wellbeing, they may feel encouraged to join you which will set your future up to have behavior spotters and lifetime friends that have the same problems as you. In fact, why not ask the people you care about to join you on this seven-day journey?

Your time is now, so let's make it count.

Day 1 and 2

Set a daily schedule for the next two days to include:
   - Get up no later than eight in the morning

- Eat breakfast; even if you feel nauseous, force yourself to eat something bland such as toast

and an apple.

- Drink a cup of herbal tea on your own, in the quiet (preferably outside) and repeat your

chosen daily affirmations.

- If you live with someone, hug them for longer than five seconds.

- Shower. ALWAYS.

- No later than eleven in the morning, do some exercise for fifteen minutes. See chapter five.

- After exercise repeat three times 'By exercising I am on my way to contentment'.

- Relaxation activity for at least thirty minutes (see suggestions below).

- No later than one in the afternoon, eat lunch.

- After lunch, journal and gratitude with herbal tea and a snack (any kind of treat).

- No later than three in the afternoon, call a friend for 15 mins – even if you don't want to. Talk about anything except how you are feeling (you need a distraction from your feelings right now).

- Relaxation activity for at least thirty minutes, with a snack. The snack is really important! Don't skip it!

- No later than six in the evening, eat dinner.

- At seven in the evening, bath – repeat daily affirmations during your bath.

- At eight in the evening, after your bath, meditate for 5 minutes. Maybe try the headspace app?

- At ten in the evening, crawl into bed and read for thirty minutes. If you can't sleep, try some of the tips in Chapter 5.

What is relaxing for you?

Suggestions; reading, listening to music, watching TV, walking, painting, word search puzzles, baking.

DAY 3 and 4

- Get up no later than eight in the morning.

- Eat breakfast and drink herbal tea while journaling.

- Shower. Ideally use some aromatherapy oils in the bathroom while showering.

- No later than ten in the morning, do some exercise outside. See chapter five.

- After exercise repeat three times 'By exercising, I am on my way to peace and strength"

- Only if you really feel you need to, check in with work to reassure yourself they have not collapsed without you!

- No later than one in the afternoon, eat lunch.

- After lunch, yoga or breathing exercises. See chapter six.

- No later than three in the afternoon, call a friend and chat for fifteen minutes or more.

- Relaxation activity for at least thirty minutes with a snack.

- No later than six in the evening, eat dinner and consider what you are grateful for today.

- At seven in the evening, have a bath, repeat daily affirmations.

- At eight in the evening, 5-minute meditation practice or use the headspace app.

- At ten in the evening, crawl into bed and read for thirty minutes.

DAY 5 and 6

- Get up no later than eight in the morning.

- Eat breakfast and drink herbal tea while journaling.

- Shower.

- No later than ten in the morning, do some exercise for thirty minutes outside. See chapter five.

- After exercise, repeat three times 'By exercising, I am clearing my mind and strengthening my body.'

- No later than one in the afternoon, eat lunch.

- After lunch, watch an uplifting film.

- No later than three in the afternoon, call a friend for fifteen minutes or longer.

- Relaxation activity for at least thirty minutes with a snack.

- No later than six in the evening, eat dinner and review your previous journaling. Do you feel the same?

- Yoga or stretching for 15 minutes and repeat daily affirmations.

- At eight in the evening, 5 minutes meditation.

- At ten in the evening, read for thirty minutes, preferably in bed.

Day 7

- Wake up no later than eight in the morning.

- Be mindful while eating breakfast and journaling.

- Shower and play your favorite music while getting dressed.

- By ten in the morning, do some light exercises such as stretching, or yoga.

- Sit or take a walk outside and make a note of the sounds you hear around you.

- While being outside, repeat 'By going outside, I am refreshing my mind and investing in wellbeing.'

- No later than one in the afternoon, eat lunch.

- Call a friend and talk to them about your 7-day experience.

- Enjoy some out-of-the-moment breathing for 5 minutes. See chapter six.

- Write down 3 new affirmations that resonate with you right now.

- During dinner, make a mental note of 3 things you are grateful for today.

- After dinner spend 30 minutes writing down how you feel at the end of the 7 days. Do you feel calmer? Do you feel energized? Maybe you feel bored!

- At eight in the evening, meditate and consider creating a weekly meditation plan for yourself.

- At ten at night, take yourself to bed and congratulate yourself for investing this time in your health and wellbeing. Consider what you have learned during this week and what you can continue to do on a regular basis.

THANK YOU NOTE

To all of you who are suffering, and have tried
to find answers through reading my book,
I wish you patience and strength. Thank
you for seeking help through my words
and know that I understand how
debilitating anxiety and panic can feel.
Remember, that as long as you are
dedicated to change, and committed to
overcoming your anxiety, you will find the
strength and power to do so. For me to
finally overcome my anxiety I needed to
believe in myself, and now, I am going to
believe in you. Through this book I want
you to know, you are not alone, and you
will get through the present challenges and
any future obstacles that come your way.

— TORI WARNER

RESOURCES

- *Bhargava, H. (2020, June 25). Anxiety Disorders: Types, Causes, Symptoms, Diagnosis, Treatment. Retrieved October 13, 2020, from https://www.webmd.com/anxiety-panic/guide/anxiety-disorders*
- *(2018, December 19). Retrieved October 13, 2020, from https://www.nhs.uk/conditions/generalised-anxiety-disorder/*
- *Post Traumatic Stress Disorder. (2020, August 14). Retrieved October 13, 2020, from https://www.anxietycanada.com/disorders/post-traumatic-stress-disorder/*
- *Smith, K., PhD. (2019, September 06). Grief and Anxiety: Complicated Grief to Anxiety Disorder.*

Retrieved October 13, 2020, from
https://www.psycom.net/anxiety-complicated-grief/

- Holland, K. (2020, March 28). *What Triggers Anxiety? 11 Causes That May Surprise you.* Retrieved October 13, 2020, from https://www.healthline.com/health/anxiety/anxiety-triggers#1

- *Causes of anxiety.* (n.d.). Retrieved October 13, 2020, from https://www.mind.org.uk/information-support/types-of-mental-health-problems/anxiety-and-panic-attacks/causes-of-anxiety/

- *Nature vs. Nurture Debate.* (2018, September 28). Retrieved October 13, 2020, from https://www.goodtherapy.org/blog/psychpedia/nature-versus-nurture

- Caraballo, J. (2018, April 17). *Is Anxiety Genetic?* Retrieved October 13, 2020, from https://www.talkspace.com/blog/is-anxiety-genetic/

- Ankrom, S. (2019, July 15). *Research Suggests Biological Cause of Panic Disorder.* Retrieved October 13, 2020, from https://www.verywellmind.com/biological-theories-of-panic-disorder-2583924

- Meek, W. (2020, February 07). *How Learned Helplessness Can Make Things Seem Impossible.* Retrieved October 13, 2020, from https://www.verywellmind.com/learned-helplessness-1393027

- *The Vicious Cycle of Anxiety.* (n.d.). Retrieved

October 13, 2020, from https://www.cci.health.wa.gov.au/-/media/CCI/Mental-Health-Professionals/Panic/Panic---Information-Sheets/Panic-Information-Sheet---03---The-Vicious-Cycle-of-Anxiety.pdf

- *Amygdala. (n.d.). Retrieved October 13, 2020, from https://www.unlearninganxiety.com/amygdala*
- *Feeling Impulsive Or Overly Emotional? Here Are 3 Proven Ways To Calm Down An Overactive Amygdala. (2020, May 06). Retrieved October 13, 2020, from https://www.calmwithyoga.com/feeling-impulsive-or-overly-emotional-here-are-3-proven-ways-to-calm-down-an-overactive-amygdala/*
- *McLaughlin, K., Rith-Najarian, L., Dirks, M., & Sheridan, M. (2013, October 24). Low vagal tone magnifies the association between psychosocial stress exposure and internalizing psychopathology in adolescents. Retrieved October 13, 2020, from https://www.ncbi.nlm.nih.gov/pmc/ articles/PMC4076387/*
- *Fallix, J. (2017, January 21). How to Stimulate your Vagus Nerve for Better Mental Health. Retrieved October 13, 2020, from https://sass.uottawa.ca/sites/ sass.uottawa.ca/files/ how_to_stimulate_your_vagus_nerve_for_better_ mental_health_1.pdf*
- *Walling, S. (2018, November 16). How to Hack Your Own Vagus Nerve. Retrieved October 13, 2020,*

from https://zenfounder.com/managing-stress/hacking-the-system-what-you-need-to-know-about-the-vagus-nerve/

- *Publishing, H. (2020, July 6). Understanding the stress response. Retrieved October 13, 2020, from https://www.health.harvard.edu/staying-healthy/understanding-the-stress-response*
- *Beware High Levels of Cortisol, the Stress Hormone. (2017, February 5). Retrieved October 13, 2020, from https://www.premierhealth.com/your-health/articles/women-wisdom-wellness-/beware-high-levels-of-cortisol-the-stress-hormone*
- *Cafasso, J. (2018, November 01). Adrenaline Rush: Everything You Should Know. Retrieved October 13, 2020, from https://www.healthline.com/health/adrenaline-rush#how-to-control*
- *Adrenaline. (2018, January). Retrieved October 13, 2020, from https://www.yourhormones.info/hormones/adrenaline/*
- *Klein, S. (2013, April 19). Adrenaline, Cortisol, Norepinephrine: The Three Major Stress Hormones. Retrieved October 13, 2020, from https://www.huffingtonpost.ca/entry/adrenaline-cortisol-stress-hormones_n_3112800*
- *Justin. (2019, September 03). Get rid of sleep anxiety and insomnia: Your guide to a better night's rest. Retrieved October 13, 2020, from*

https://www.stress.org/get-rid-of-sleep-anxiety-and-insomnia-your-guide-to-a-better-nights-rest

- Jennings, K. (2018, August 28). *16 Simple Ways to Relieve Stress and Anxiety.* Retrieved October 13, 2020, from https://www.healthline.com/nutrition/16-ways-relieve-stress-anxiety

- Julson, E. (2018, May 10). *10 Best Ways to Increase Dopamine Levels Naturally.* Retrieved October 13, 2020, from https://www.healthline.com/nutrition/how-to-increase-dopamine

- Tremblay, S. (2018, December 06). *Can Vitamin B Raise Serotonin?* Retrieved October 13, 2020, from https://healthyeating.sfgate.com/can-vitamin-b-raise-serotonin-5975.html

- Korb, A., PhD. (2011, November 17). *Boosting Your Serotonin Activity.* Retrieved October 13, 2020, from https://www.psychologytoday.com/ca/blog/prefrontal-nudity/201111/boosting-your-serotonin-activity

- Naoumidis, Alex. *Thinking Traps: 12 Cognitive Distortions That Are Hijacking Your Brain.* 22 Nov. 2019, www.mindsethealth.com/matter/thinking-traps-cognitive-distortions.

- "Thinking Traps." *Anxiety Canada,* 11 Sept. 2019, www.anxietycanada.com/articles/thinking-traps/.

- Clear, James. "The 3 R's of Habit Change: How To Start New Habits That Actually Stick." *Jamesclear,*

13 Nov. 2018, jamesclear.com/three-steps-habit-change.

- Moore, Catherine. "Positive Daily Affirmations: Is There Science Behind It?" PositivePsychology.com, 13 Oct. 2020, positivepsychology.com/daily-affirmations/.
- Tams, L. (2018, September 20). Journaling to reduce stress. MSU Extension. https://www.canr.msu.edu/news/journaling_to_reduce_stress.
- Robinson, L. The Mental Health Benefits of Exercise. HelpGuide.org. https://www.helpguide.org/articles/healthy-living/the-mental-health-benefits-of-exercise.htm.
- Ratey, J. J. (2019, October 22). Can exercise help treat anxiety? Harvard Health Blog. https://www.health.harvard.edu/blog/can-exercise-help-treat-anxiety-2019102418096.
- Wolff, C. (2019, July 29). 6 Habits That Help You Commit to a Workout Routine. Aaptiv. https://aaptiv.com/magazine/commit-to-a-workout-routine.
- Robinson, L. How to Start Exercising and Stick to It. HelpGuide.org. https://www.helpguide.org/articles/healthy-living/how-to-start-exercising-and-stick-to-it.htm.
- U.S. Department of Health and Human Services. Sleep Deprivation and Deficiency. National Heart Lung and Blood Institute.

https://www.nhlbi.nih.gov/health-topics/sleep-deprivation-and-deficiency.

- Green, E. (2020, February 7). *A Bedtime Routine For Adults: 10 Relaxing Activities For Sleep*. No Sleepless Nights. https://www.nosleeplessnights.com/sleep-hygiene/bedtime-routine-for-adults/.

- Fiorenzi, R. (2020, October 4). *Best Essential Oils for Sleep and Insomnia*. Start Sleeping. https://startsleeping.org/best-essential-oils-for-sleep-and-insomnia/.

- Schildhouse, J. (2020, September 29). *9 Best Vitamins for Sleep*. The Healthy. https://www.thehealthy.com/nutrition/vitamins/best-vitamins-for-sleep/.

- Robinson02, J. (2019, May 2). *Natural Sleep Aids & Supplements*. WebMD. https://www.webmd.com/sleep-disorders/ss/slideshow-natural-sleep-remedies.

- *Abdominal Breathing*. guysandthomas. (2016, January). https://www.guysandstthomas.nhs.uk/resources/patient-information/therapies/abdominal-breathing.pdf.

- Gotter, A. (2020, June 17). *Box Breathing*. Healthline. https://www.healthline.com/health/box-breathing.

- *4 – 7 – 8 Breath Relaxation Exercise*. Cordem. (2010, February).

https://www.cordem.org/globalassets/files/academic-assembly/2017-aa/handouts/day-three/biofeedback-exercises-for-stress-2---fernances-j.pdf.

- *Stop Anxiety In Its Tracks With This Move. The Yoga School – A sanctuary in the sky. (2018, November 12). https://yogaschool.asia/stop-anxiety-in-its-tracks-with-this-move/.*

- *Bubnis, D. (2020, October 2). Which Type of Meditation Is Right for Me? healthline. https://www.healthline.com/health/mental-health/types-of-meditation#mindfulness-meditation.*

- *The science-backed benefits of daily meditation. Headspace. https://www.headspace.com/meditation/daily-meditation.*

- *8 reasons why you don't stick with new habits (and how to stick with them). Habits Buzz. (2019, November 21). https://habitsbuzz.com/how-stick-with-new-habits/.*

- *Good habits take time: how to deal with failure and falling off the wagon. The Monk Life. (2017, May 9). https://www.themonklife.net/good-habits-take-time/.*

- *Clear, J. (2020, February 4). How to Get Back on Track: 7 Ways to Bounce Back After Slipping Up. James Clear. https://jamesclear.com/get-back-on-track.*

- *Skarnulis, L. (2010, September 28). 10 Easy Ways to Make Exercise a Habit. WebMD.*

https://www.webmd.com/women/features/exercise-habits.

- *U.S. National Library of Medicine. (2020, April 9). Changing your sleep habits: MedlinePlus Medical Encyclopedia. MedlinePlus. https://medlineplus.gov/ency/ patientinstructions/000757.htm.*

- *Anxiety vs. Anxiety Disorders. ULifeline. http://www.ulifeline.org/articles/439-anxiety-vs-anxiety-disorders.*

- *Ho, T. (2020, March 14). How to Put Yourself First? Your Ultimate Self Care Guide. Happy Free Lifestyle. https://happyfreelifestyle.com/personal-growth/putyourselffirst/.*

- *4 ways to boost your self-compassion. Harvard Health. https://www.health.harvard.edu/mental-health/4-ways-to-boost-your-self-compassion.*

- *Raypole, C. (2019, April 22). 6 Ways to Boost Serotonin Without Medication. healthline. https://www.healthline.com/health/how-to-increase-serotonin.*

NOTES

1. WHAT THE HECK IS ANXIETY ANYWAY?

1. · Bhargava, H. (2020, June 25). Anxiety Disorders: Types, Causes, Symptoms, Diagnosis, Treatment. Retrieved October 13, 2020, from https://www.webmd.com/anxiety-panic/guide/anxiety-disorders

2. · (2018, December 19). Retrieved October 13, 2020, from https://www.nhs.uk/conditions/generalised-anxiety-disorder/

3. Causes of anxiety. (n.d.). Retrieved October 13, 2020, from https://www.mind.org.uk/information-support/types-of-mental-health-problems/anxiety-and-panic-attacks/causes-of-anxiety/

4. Holland, K. (2020, March 28). What Triggers Anxiety? 11 Causes That May Surprise you. Retrieved October 13, 2020, from https://www.healthline.com/health/anxiety/anxiety-triggers#1

5. Nature vs. Nurture Debate. (2018, September 28). Retrieved October 13, 2020, from https://www.goodtherapy.org/blog/psychpedia/nature-versus-nurture

6. Ankrom, S. (2019, July 15). Research Suggests Biological Cause of Panic Disorder. Retrieved October 13, 2020, from https://www.verywell-mind.com/biological-theories-of-panic-disorder-2583924

7. The Vicious Cycle of Anxiety. (n.d.). Retrieved October 13, 2020, from https://www.cci.health.wa.gov.au/-/media/CCI/Mental-Health-Professionals/Panic/Panic---Information-Sheets/Panic-Information-Sheet---03---The-Vicious-Cycle-of-Anxiety.pdf

8. Post Traumatic Stress Disorder. (2020, August 14). Retrieved October 13, 2020, from https://www.anxietycanada.com/disorders/post-traumatic-stress-disorder/

9. Smith, K., PhD. (2019, September 06). Grief and Anxiety: Complicated Grief to Anxiety Disorder. Retrieved October 13, 2020, from https://www.psycom.net/anxiety-complicated-grief/

2. BASIC (AND I MEAN BASIC) BRAIN BIOLOGY

1. Amygdala. (n.d.). Retrieved October 13, 2020, from https://www.un-learninganxiety.com/amygdala

2. Feeling Impulsive Or Overly Emotional? Here Are 3 Proven Ways To Calm Down An Overactive Amygdala. (2020, May 06). Retrieved October 13, 2020, from https://www.calmwithyoga.com/feeling-impulsive-or-overly-emotional-here-are-3-proven-ways-to-calm-down-an-overactive-amygdala/

3. McLaughlin, K., Rith-Najarian, L., Dirks, M., & Sheridan, M. (2013, October 24). Low vagal tone magnifies the association between psychosocial stress exposure and internalizing psychopathology in adolescents. Retrieved October 13, 2020, from https://www.ncbi.nlm.nih.gov/pmc/articles/PMC4076387/

   Walling, S. (2018, November 16). How to Hack Your Own Vagus Nerve. Retrieved October 13, 2020, from https://zenfounder.com/managing-stress/hacking-the-system-what-you-need-to-know-about-the-vagus-nerve/

4. Fallix, J. (2017, January 21). How to Stimulate your Vagus Nerve for Better Mental Health. Retrieved October 13, 2020, from https://sass.uottawa.ca/sites/sass.uottawa.ca/files/how_to_stimulate_your_vagus_nerve_for_better_mental_health_1.pdf

3. HORMONES AND STRESS

1. Beware High Levels of Cortisol, the Stress Hormone. (2017, February 5). Retrieved October 13, 2020, from https://www.premierhealth.com/your-health/articles/women-wisdom-wellness-/beware-high-levels-of-cortisol-the-stress-hormone

2. Publishing, H. (2020, July 6). Understanding the stress response. Retrieved October 13, 2020, from https://www.health.harvard.edu/staying-healthy/understanding-the-stress-response

3. Adrenaline. (2018, January). Retrieved October 13, 2020, from https://www.yourhormones.info/hormones/adrenaline/

4. Cafasso, J. (2018, November 01). Adrenaline Rush: Everything You

Should Know. Retrieved October 13, 2020, from https://www.health-line.com/health/adrenaline-rush#how-to-control

5. Justin. (2019, September 03). Get rid of sleep anxiety and insomnia: Your guide to a better night's rest. Retrieved October 13, 2020, from https://www.stress.org/get-rid-of-sleep-anxiety-and-insomnia-your-guide-to-a-better-nights-rest

6. Julson, E. (2018, May 10). 10 Best Ways to Increase Dopamine Levels Naturally. Retrieved October 13, 2020, from https://www.healthline.-com/nutrition/how-to-increase-dopamine

7. Tremblay, S. (2018, December 06). Can Vitamin B Raise Serotonin? Retrieved October 13, 2020, from https://healthyeating.sfgate.com/can-vitamin-b-raise-serotonin-5975.html

8. Raypole, C. (2019, April 22). *6 Ways to Boost Serotonin Without Medication.* healthline. https://www.healthline.com/health/how-to-increase-serotonin.

4. SELF-TALK AND JOURNALING

1. Moore, Catherine. "Positive Daily Affirmations: Is There Science Behind It?" *PositivePsychology.com*, 13 Oct. 2020, positivepsychology.com/daily-affirmations/.

2. *8 reasons why you don't stick with new habits (and how to stick with them).* Habits Buzz. (2019, November 21). https://habitsbuzz.com/how-stick-with-new-habits/.

3. Clear, James. "The 3 R's of Habit Change: How To Start New Habits That Actually Stick." *Jamesclear*, 13 Nov. 2018, jamesclear.com/three-steps-habit-change.

4. Naoumidis, Alex. *Thinking Traps: 12 Cognitive Distortions That Are Hijacking Your Brain.* 22 Nov. 2019, www.-mindsethealth.com/matter/thinking-traps-cognitive-distortions.

5. Tams, L. (2018, September 20). *Journaling to reduce stress.* MSU Extension. https://www.canr.msu.edu/news/journaling_to_reduce_stress.

5. WHY EXERCISE AND SLEEP SHOULD BE
TOP OF OUR TO-DO LISTS

1. Robinson, L. *The Mental Health Benefits of Exercise.*
   HelpGuide.org.
   https://www.helpguide.org/articles/healthy-living/the-mental-health-benefits-of-exercise.htm.
   Ratey, J. J. (2019, October 22). *Can exercise help treat anxiety?*
   Harvard Health Blog.
   https://www.health.harvard.edu/blog/can-exercise-help-treat-anxiety-2019102418096.
2. Wolff, C. (2019, July 29). *6 Habits That Help You Commit to a Workout Routine.*
   Aaptiv. https://aaptiv.com/magazine/commit-to-a-workout-routine.
3. U.S. Department of Health and Human Services. *Sleep Deprivation and Deficiency.* National Heart Lung and Blood Institute.
   https://www.nhlbi.nih.gov/health-topics/sleep-deprivation-and-deficiency.
4. Green, E. (2020, February 7). *A Bedtime Routine For Adults: 10 Relaxing Activities For Sleep.* No Sleepless Nights. https://www.nosleeplessnights.com/sleep-hygiene/bedtime-routine-for-adults/.
5. Fiorenzi, R. (2020, October 4). *Best Essential Oils for Sleep and Insomnia.*
   Start Sleeping.
   https://startsleeping.org/best-essential-oils-for-sleep-and-insomnia/.

6. BREATHING – IN THE MOMENT AND
OUT OF THE MOMENT

1. *Abdominal Breathing.* guysandthomas. (2016, January).
   https://www.guysandstthomas.nhs.uk/resources/patient-information/therapies/abdominal-breathing.pdf.

2. Gotter, A. (2020, June 17). *Box Breathing*. Healthline. https://www.healthline.com/health/box-breathing.

3. *4 – 7 – 8 Breath Relaxation Exercise.* Cordem. (2010, February). https://www.cordem.org/globalassets/files/academic-assembly/2017-aa/handouts/day-three/biofeedback-exercises-for-stress-2---fernances-j.pdf.

4. Bubnis, D. (2020, October 2). *Which Type of Meditation Is Right for Me?* healthline. https://www.healthline.com/health/mental-health/types-of-meditation#mindfulness-meditation.

5. *The science-backed benefits of daily meditation.* Headspace. https://www.headspace.com/meditation/daily-meditation.

7. COMMIT TO LONG-TERM HABITS

1. *Good habits take time: how to deal with failure and falling off the wagon.* The Monk Life. (2017, May 9). https://www.themonklife.net/good-habits-take-time/.

   Clear, J. (2020, February 4). *How to Get Back on Track: 7 Ways to Bounce Back After Slipping Up.* James Clear. https://jamesclear.com/get-back-on-track.

2. Raypole, C. (2019, April 22). *6 Ways to Boost Serotonin Without Medication.* healthline. https://www.healthline.com/health/how-to-increase-serotonin.

3. Skarnulis, L. (2010, September 28). *10 Easy Ways to Make Exercise a Habit.* WebMD. https://www.webmd.com/women/features/exercise-habits.

4. U.S. National Library of Medicine. (2020, April 9). *Changing your sleep habits: MedlinePlus Medical Encyclopedia.* MedlinePlus. https://medlineplus.gov/ency/patientinstructions/000757.htm.

8. PULLING IT ALL TOGETHER

1. Ho, T. (2020, March 14). *How to Put Yourself First? Your Ultimate Self Care Guide*. Happy Free Lifestyle. https://happyfreelifestyle.com/personal-growth/putyourselffirst/.
2. Korb, A., PhD. (2011, November 17). Boosting Your Serotonin Activity. Retrieved October 13, 2020, from https://www.psychologytoday.com/ca/blog/prefrontal-nudity/201111/boosting-your-serotonin-activity

Printed in Great Britain
by Amazon